Theory and Nursing
a systematic approach

Theory and Nursing

a systematic approach

Peggy L. Chinn, RN, PhD, FAAN

Director, Graduate Nursing Programs,
Research Professor of Nursing,
Center for Human Caring,
University of Colorado,
Denver, Colorado

Maeona K. Kramer, RN, PhD

Professor of Nursing
University of Utah,
Salt Lake City, Utah

THIRD EDITION

with 23 illustrations

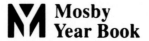

Mosby
Year Book

St. Louis   Baltimore   Boston   Chicago   London   Philadelphia   Sydney   Toronto

1991

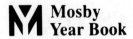

Mosby
Year Book

Dedicated to Publishing Excellence

Editor: N. Darlene Como
Developmental editor: Laurie Sparks
Project manager: Patricia Gayle May
Production editor: Mary Cusick Drone
Designer: Susan Lane

THIRD EDITION

Printed in the United States of America
Mosby-Year Book, Inc.
11830 Westline Industrial Drive
St. Louis, MO 63146

Library of Congress Cataloging-in-Publication Data

Chinn, Peggy L.
    Theory and nursing : a systematic approach / Peggy L. Chinn,
Maeona K. Kramer. — 3rd ed.
       p.   cm.
    Includes bibliographical references.
    Includes index.
    ISBN 0-8016-0970-4
    1. Nursing—Philosophy.   I. Kramer, Maeona K.   II. Title.
    [DNLM: 1. Nursing Theory.   WY 86 C539t]
    RT84.5.C49   1991
    610.73′01—dc20
    DNLM/DLC
    for Library of Congress   90-636
                                                                     CIP

UG/DC   9   8   7   6   5   4   3   2   1

Preface

Countless circumstances have prompted the nature of the revisions to this third edition. These include dialogue with colleagues throughout the world, challenges to our personal values, emerging feminist theory, critical examination of our previous writings, and shifts in nursing and health care. This edition follows directly from criticisms of students and faculty who used the first and second editions, as well as our own critical thinking in response to those criticisms. Some of the material in previous editions was interpreted in ways we had not intended; other responses reflected consistent understandings of our intents, but our intents have shifted drastically. All of the discussion around these issues has jolted us to new levels of awareness. We quickly discovered how radically our thinking has changed and how deep the changes in our profession flow.

The dramatic shifts in nursing that have influenced our revision include:
- the diverse forms of scholarship that are valued for the discipline,
- the emerging clarity concerning the ethic of caring that informs the philosophic underpinnings of the discipline, and
- the central role of nursing in the context of the current health care system crisis.

These shifts form a context that supports a perspective that seeks liberation from, rather than perpetuation of, the status quo. This edition of the book builds on the traditional views that we presented in the first and second editions, but moves beyond the limitations inherent in those views. We constructed the content of this book to open the way for challenge and criticism of current practices around theory and knowledge.

The most dramatic and pervasive shift in this edition is in the language. Our initial aim with respect to the language of this edition was to shift the writing style to a clearer, more accessible, and more readable form. We have always maintained as a basic premise of the book that theory and practice need to "connect" with one another. Consistent with this commitment we began the editing process with the intent to eliminate words and phrases that depended on or assumed a style typically reserved for the advanced academician. We began by simplifying the sentence structure, eliminating pretentious words when a common word would do, shifting to the active voice as much as possible, and limiting the use of pronouns to instances when an agent is clearly identifiable. As we worked, we became aware of more "flaws" in the underlying structure of the language and tried to address them as consistently as possible. We became conscious of value assumptions and connotations that were inherent in the language. Many of the terms that are commonly associated with the practice of scientific methods carry antagonistic, adversarial, objectifying, and militaristic connotations that are contrary to the intents of an ethic of caring and new views of human science. The term "whip lines" (now wave lines) is an example of a term that was built into our conception of the system for theory development. Other terms that we found to occur with impressive frequency were terms and phrases like "competing images," "judgments," "capture," "aim," "target," "operation," "boundaries," "argument," and "debate." Even when the strict meaning of the word was adequate for the text, we sought to shift the language to words that carry a similar literal meaning but a more human and caring value connotation. For example, instead of the phrase "argue your position," we use instead "share your ideas."

There were other subtle meanings that we had built into the language and structure of the book, some of which were contradictory to our intent, an intent that dated back to the first edition. For example, we did not intend to prescribe "set" or "best" approaches or to convey a strict adherence to linearity in thinking or in construction. Yet much of what we presented was both prescriptive and linear. In this edition we shifted from a prescriptive criteria-based approach to a mode of questioning and considering alternatives. We invite you, the reader, to explore responses to the questions, forming avenues for creating new directions. We deleted references to the "first," "second," or "third" "step" in a process, speaking instead of issues or alternatives that could be addressed in the context of a process.

Another shift that we made in the language is informed by our intent to reframe traditional relationships between people. We have sought to directly engage and empower the reader. We speak directly to the reader as "you," with the intent to empower the reader's own abilities and ideas rather than to impose the authoritative voice of the text. For example, in Chapter 5 we speak of how model cases are used in forming conceptual meaning by stating: "When you consider your model case placed in several different social contexts, you create an avenue for perceiving important values and make deliberate choices concerning them."

In essence, this edition of the book has been completely rewritten. Much of the content is similar, so that it is still recognizable as the same book. However, the shifts in the language are profound. The shifts set the stage for further movement toward new methods in nursing and are consistent with fundamental philosophic shifts in nursing that will ultimately change the development and expression of knowledge.

Preface

The following paragraphs describe the structural and content revisions that we have made:

Chapter 1 now focuses exclusively on nursing's patterns of knowing. (The second half of this chapter in the previous edition is now Chapter 2.) We revised the presentation of the patterns of knowing to achieve greater clarity and simplicity. We revised some of the language that we used to describe the patterns and methods associated with the patterns and tried to reduce connotations of linearity and categorizations that are associated with the patterns. We clarified the distinction between "empirics" as it applies to nursing's pattern of knowing, and "traditional science," which we have used to describe methods of science that draw on many of the assumptions of empirics. A fundamental shift that we made in this section is the move toward increasing integration of all of the patterns. We no longer see esthetics as both a pattern and a means of integration, but rather we see integration as an essential process in the wholeness of knowing. Integration necessarily grows out of the use of any of the methods that are unique to a particular pattern.

Chapter 2, formerly the second half of Chapter 1, now focuses on theory as the expression of empirics. We made dramatic shifts in our conceptions of empiric theory and how it is developed based on the idea of integrating more fully the philosophic perspectives of the whole of knowing within the processes of any one pattern. For example, rather than using the idea of "concept analysis" in the system for theory development, we shifted to the idea of "creating conceptual meaning." Here, the process becomes less mechanistic and prescribed and more innovative, imaginative, and creative. Some of the same "procedures" are described for this process, but they are now presented as suggested tools to explore possible meanings in the overall process of creating a meaning for a particular purpose. Other processes are described in ways that open possibilities for drawing on all patterns of knowing to create a more whole, or fuller understanding.

Chapter 3 (formerly Chapter 2) focuses on the historic emergence of the key concepts of the discipline. We eliminated the long and awkward table in the second edition, using instead four tables that summarize the evolution of key theoretic ideas around the nursing concepts of person, environment, society, and nursing. We added some of the ideas that were previously part of Chapter 9, to show a chronology of the evolving directions in theory during the first 30 years of formal theory development in nursing. This chapter focuses on theory development through the early 1980s. We discuss shifts that emerged in the 1980s when nurse scholars began to focus on the development of research and theory at a midrange level, more specifically addressing problems and phenomenon that are located within nursing's scope of practice and the health and illness experience of people who receive nursing care.

Chapter 4 (formerly Chapter 3) now reflects the shifts that have emerged in nursing concerning what types of theory and philosophy or ethic is required for practice. We retained a description of four definitions of theory presented in nursing literature, substituting in this edition Jean Watson's definition instead of the definition of Barbara Stevens. The Watson definition addresses explicitly the creative and imaginative dimensions that are required for human science theory. We made a dramatic shift in our own definition of theory, which is now "a creative and rigorous structuring of ideas that project a tentative, purposeful, and systematic view of phenomena." Our previous definition was "a set of concepts, definition, and propositions that projects a systematic view of phenomena by designating specific interrelationships among concepts for purposes of describing, explaining, and predicting phenomena." One shift that is most dramatic is the move away from the teleologic (outcome focused) purposes of traditional science (description, explanation, and prediction) as definitive for theory. The new definition places the theorist at the center; it defines theory in a way that the theorist's own creativity is central in structuring a particular view stated as theory. The new definition also emphasizes the tentative nature of theory, which in turn affects conceptions of what theory is useful for.

Chapter 5 (formerly Chapter 4) fills in the details of how the various components of the processes for theory development emerge. The process of creating conceptual meaning (formerly called concept analysis) includes the activities that we described earlier (for example, examining definition, building cases), but we revised these to reflect ideas of thinking and rethinking. We also draw on additional sources that can contribute to the formation of conceptual meaning, particularly in the arts. The process of creating conceptual meaning is conveyed as a tool to create a useful meaning rather than to prescribe a definition. We retained guidelines for forming criteria for a concept that can be used for research and practice purposes, but we have stressed the tentative nature of any definition or criteria and the fact that these are constructed to be consistent with an intended meaning for a specific purpose.

The process of structuring and contextualizing theory (formerly the construction of theoretic relationships) has assumed a major shift with respect to the idea of contextualizing. This grew out of our thinking about the boundaries of a theory, but the idea now includes the importance of the situational context in which a theory is placed, as well as the limits of its applicability. The process of generating and testing theoretic relationships (formerly testing of theoretic relationships) assumes a similar subtle but important shift. The idea of "generating" explicitly incorporates the methods of theory development that are grounded, inductive, or phenomenologic. It also emphasizes the creative, reflective component in building theoretic ideas. The process of deliberative application of theory (formerly practical validation of theory) shifts the focus to the applicability of the theory with a conscious, deliberate intent. We chose the word "deliberative" because of its use by nurse theorist Orlando, who describes "deliberative nursing actions" as those that are done with thoughtful reflection to solve and prevent problems. The process of deliberative application of theory requires a planned approach drawing on the research methods we described in previous editions, but includes the ideas of achieving quality of care and practice goals that are chosen by nurses in clinical settings.

Chapters 6 and 7 (formerly Chapters 5 and 6) focus on description (Chapter 6) and critical reflection (Chapter 7) of theory. In former editions we referred to "evaluation of theory," implying a predetermined or prescribed set of criteria by which a theory was "judged" to be "good." In this edition we shifted the emphasis in both chapters to the process of asking questions and exploring various responses to those questions. By doing so, the processes become fluid and amenable to situational considerations that only the reader can fully appreciate. We provide suggestions and guidelines for achieving a complete, sound, and thorough description of theory and for taking a position with respect to a theory's value for the reader's purpose. The questions shift away from predetermined "facts" or "criteria" by which theory is described and judged to a focus on the reader's own intent with respect to the theory, examination of that intent, and building responses that clarify and communicate the reader's ideas about the theory.

Chapters 8 and 9 (formerly Chapters 7 and 8) remain similar to those in the second edition. In Chapter 8, which focuses on the links between theory and research, we updated the example of a theory-testing research study. In Chapter 9, which focuses on links between theory and practice, we changed the content to be consistent with the changes in conceptualizing deliberative application of theory and added a section on the use of theory to achieve quality of care standards in practice. Both of these chapters retain the strong features of the previous editions in providing specific guidelines for strengthening the theory-practice-research links.

The new *appendix* in this edition was the former Chapter 9 in the first and second editions, which consisted of a brief overview of the essential ideas proposed by the early nurse theorists. We included and updated these overviews for this appendix. This material now represents a summary of the early theoretic writings in nursing that predate the shifts in nursing theory away from the grand or general theories (which these are) to a midrange, practice-

and-research–based form of theorizing in nursing. We do not intend this appendix to provide a comprehensive summary of nursing's theoretic writings, nor do we intend it to reflect the most recent developments in nursing theory. We retained these summaries in this form because of their historic significance and because of their continuing usefulness in guiding new theoretic work, for building curricula, and for designing nursing care systems.

The *glossary* and *bibliography* have been revised and updated. The glossary retains its style and form, providing page references to discussions in the text. It has been revised to be consistent with the language shifts in the text. We updated the bibliography to delete references that are no longer useful in the study of theory development and added recent references that are pertinent to theory development and shifts in philosphy and method that inform activities of theory development.

As with any endeavor of this scope, it has not been accomplished alone. Specifically, we want to thank Dr. Linda K. Amos and Dr. Sue Huether for valuing this scholarly work. They provided the time and resources that we needed to see it to completion, including making it possible for us to be together geographically. Charlene Eldridge helped us with word processing and editing in the eleventh hour and provided significant guidance in bringing the problems of language to our conscious awareness. Barbara Carper has engaged in many discussions with us that helped to clarify and inform our thinking with respect to nursing's patterns of knowing. Students who have participated in our theory classes at the University of Utah and at the State University of New York at Buffalo challenged our thinking and provided the ground from which we developed important insights. We are indebted to reviewers of our writings that have appeared in journals over the past 5 years, many of whom are anonymous, as well as authors of journal articles that have criticized our work. Our close friends and families have now lived through this process three times, and we are lovingly grateful for their continuing support and the cohesiveness they provide us. Finally, we wish to acknowledge that we have not only lived through this process together three times, but that our friendship and appreciation of one another has grown immensely. Working together in this process has been a challenge and a source of growth, and the spirit in which we have worked together has made it a rewarding task both personally and professionally. We acknowledge our appreciation for one another.

Peggy L. Chinn
Maeona K. Kramer

Contents in Brief

1
Nursing's patterns of knowing, 1

2
Nursing theory as an expression of empirics, 19

3
Emergence of nursing theory, 33

4
Nursing theory: an examination of the concept, 57

5
Development of nursing theory, 79

6
Description of nursing theory, 107

7
Critical reflection of nursing theory, 127

8
Nursing theory and research, 141

9
Nursing theory and practice, 161

Appendix, 175
Glossary, 196
Bibliography, 204

Contents

1   **Nursing's patterns of knowing,** 1

How do we know? 2
The whole of knowing, 5
    Empirics: the science of nursing, 7
    Ethics: moral knowledge in nursing, 8
    Personal knowing in nursing, 9
    Esthetics: the art of nursing, 10
Processes for forming understanding, 11
Integration, 14
Patterns gone wild, 15
Conclusion, 16

2   **Nursing theory as an expression of empirics,** 19

What is theory? 20
Why does nursing need theory? 21
    Theory and professional identity, 22
    Theory and coherence of purpose, 23
    Theory and professional communication, 25
    What kind of theory? 26
How does a discipline acquire theory? 26
    Processes for theory development, 27
    The heritage of history, 28
    Wave lines, 28
    Quadrant lines, 28
    Boundary lines, 30
Use of the processes for theory development, 30
Conclusion, 31

3   **Emergence of nursing theory,** 33

History of theory development, 34
    Conceptual models and philosophies of practice, 39
    Theories borrowed from other disciplines, 40
    The development of theory within the discipline, 41
Major views expressed in early nursing models, 41
    Nature of nursing, 41
    The person, 42
    Society and environment, 45
    Health, 45

Contents

The discipline of nursing: philosophy of development of nursing
knowledge, 46
    The nature of key nursing concepts and holism, 47
The contexts of theory development, 48
    Values, 48
    Resources, 50
Evolving directions in nursing theory, 51
Conclusion, 54

4   **Nursing theory: an examination of the concept,** 57

Complexity of abstract concepts, 58
    Defining and understanding concepts, 61
    Ambiguities in definitions, 62
Comparative analysis of definitions of theory, 62
    Rose McKay: The form of theory development, 63
    James Dickoff and Patricia James: The outcome of theory, 68
    Jean Watson: The tentative nature of theory, 70
    Rosemary Ellis: Theory as a guide for inquiry, 71
A comprehensive definition of theory for nursing, 71
Definitions of terms related to theory development, 74
Conclusion, 76

5   **Development of nursing theory,** 79

Creating conceptual meaning, 80
    Selecting a concept, 83
    Clarifying your purpose, 84
    Data sources, 84
    Exploring contexts and values, 89
    Formulating criteria, 90
    Conceptual meaning and problems of theoretic development, 92
Structuring and contextualizing theory, 93
    Identifying and defining concepts, 94
    Identifying assumptions, 96
    Clarifying the context, 97
    Designing relationship statements, 98
Generating and testing theoretic relationships, 99
    Empirically grounding emerging relationships, 99
    Explicating empiric indicators, 100
    Validating relationships through empiric methods, 101
Deliberative application of theory, 102
    Selecting the clinical setting, 103
    Determining outcomes, 103
    Implementing a formal method of study, 104
Conclusion, 104

Contents

6 Description of nursing theory, 107

Components of theory, 108
Posing questions, 109
    What is the purpose of this theory? 109
    What are the concepts of this theory? 111
    How are the concepts defined? 112
    What is the nature of relationships? 113
    What is the structure of the theory? 114
    On what assumptions does the theory build? 118
    Forming a complete description, 119
Additional element of description: scope, 120
Conclusion, 125

7 Critical reflection of nursing theory, 127

Questions for reflection, 128
    How clear is this theory? 129
    How simple is this theory? 133
    How general is this theory? 134
    How accessible is this theory? 135
    How important is this theory? 136
Forming a complete critical reflection, 137
Conclusion, 137

8 Nursing theory and research, 141

Theory-linked research and isolated research, 142
    Problems of theory-linked research, 143
The relationship between theory and research, 145
    Theory-generating research, 145
    Theory-testing research, 148
Developing sound theoretic research, 149
    The clinical problem, research purpose, research problem, and
        hypotheses, 149
    Background of the study and literature review, 151
    The research method, 153
    Generalizability and usefulness of the study, 158
Conclusion, 158

9 Nursing theory and practice, 161

Creating conceptual meaning, 163
    Identification of empiric indicators, 163
    Differentiating similar concepts, 164
    Identification of new concepts, 165
    Identification of criteria for nursing diagnoses, 166

Deliberative application of theory, 167
How to determine if a theory should be applied in practice, 167
    Are the theory goals and practice goals congruous with one another?
      168
    Is the intended context of the theory congruous with the situation in
      which the theory will be applied? 169
    Is there, or might there be, similarity between theory variables and
      practice variables? 169
    Are the explanations of the theory sufficient to be used as a basis for
      nursing action? 169
    Is there research evidence supporting the theory? 170
    How will this new approach influence the practical function of the
      nursing unit? 171
Quality-related outcomes, 171
    Professional standards of care, 172
    Functional outcomes, 172
    Nurse satisfaction, 172
    Quality of care perceived by the person who receives care, 172
    Expected outcomes related to quality of life, 173
Conclusion, 173

Appendix, 175

Glossary, 196

Bibliography, 204

1
Nursing's patterns of knowing

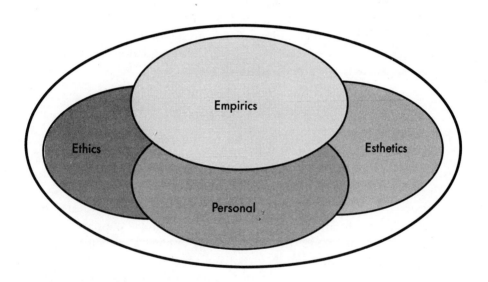

Although empiric knowledge is valuable for nursing practice, each of the patterns of knowing is essential. Each is a distinct aspect of the whole, every pattern makes a contribution to the whole, and each is equally vital.

Since Nightingale first established formal education for nurses, nursing has depended on formal knowledge as a basis for practice. The type of knowledge used in nursing has changed over the decades since Nightingale. Before 1950, nursing was viewed as a technical art that emphasized principles and procedures coupled with a spirit of unselfish devotion. By the 1950s the phrase "nursing science" began to appear in the nursing literature. Today nursing theory and research are seen as an important means of achieving scientific knowledge for nursing practice.

Although nursing science is a valuable basis for nursing practice, knowledge that does not fit the traditional definition of science is also necessary and valuable. This chapter addresses the various forms of knowing upon which nursing practice is based and provides the foundation for understanding theory as one type of nursing knowledge.

HOW DO WE KNOW?

The processes of knowing are common and fundamental human activities. Everyone, from the time of birth, begins a lifelong process of learning, of experiencing self, other people, and the environment. What people "know" is the outcome of these everyday experiences.

Processes for knowing in Western academic cultures have also been structured, formalized, and systematized. For example, Western scientists claim to know something because they have applied a particular research method or used a scientific problem-solving approach. Some nurses are educated and trained to use formalized approaches to produce structured knowledge that is known as a "body of knowledge." These nurses who are mutually engaged in producing new nursing knowledge collectively constitute and develop the "discipline" of nursing. Nurses who work in a nursing practice situation bring knowledge from lifelong learning experiences, as well as the structured knowledge of the discipline as taught through education and training.

Although various ways of knowing have been acknowledged and described in Western societies, "science" has acquired the status of a superior way for a group to develop knowledge. For example, Kerlinger identifies tenacity, authority, and a priori methods as ways of knowing that are inferior to science (Kerlinger, 1986). According to this view, tenacity is the form of knowing in which some truth is believed simply because it has always been thought to be true. Authority is a belief about what is "true" because an authoritative source or person says it is true. A priori knowing depends on reason and is not necessarily consistent with experience. These forms of knowing can all lead to the same conclusion and may even be thought of as "factual." The difference between them is in *how* one knows. For example, some people might state that sitting in a draft causes a cold. If asked how they know this is so, they might state that it "just is" (tenacity), or that their "parents said so" (authority), or that it "stands to reason" (a priori).

Knowledge about how a cold is transmitted may also be learned from the method of science. The method of science is different from tenacity, authority, or a priori ways of knowing in that empiric (experiential or sensory) observation or evidence is used as the test of whether or not something is "true." The methods of science were developed as a way to eliminate errors in judging what is actual or true by repeated tests of hypotheses or examination of research questions on the basis of empiric reality. From a scientific perspective, only that which stands the test of repeated empiric testing is thought to constitute knowledge, or truth. Therefore, if someone decided to examine whether sitting in a draft causes colds, this idea would be stated as a hypothesis and repeatedly tested to determine if empiric evidence supported the claim.

All of the forms of knowing described by Kerlinger rest on an idea about objectivity in which truth is thought to exist apart from, or outside of, the person who knows. A fundamental idea about reality from which traditional science developed is Descartian dualism, in which the rational mind and the "out there" reality of truth are viewed as separate.

A shift in ideas about the value of science as a superior way to know is emerging in nursing and society. These emerging ideas are based on a view that assumes a fundamental unity between the knower and what is known (Bleich, 1978). From this perspective, the person who perceives reality is recognized as an active participant in creating what is known. The assumption is that knowledge is created by people, and not "objectively" discovered as an "out there" reality. The emphasis is on making sense of the world in terms of the needs of the present and the future, on resolving the splits and contradictions that the traditional "objective" methods cannot resolve, and on seeking tentative understandings rather than absolute truth (Chinn, 1985).

The term "human science" has evolved in the social sciences and is used in nursing to refer to processes for empiric inquiry that account for and respect human characteristics such as motivation and intentionality. Human science methods acknowledge the effect of the scientist on what is studied. They are designed to account for the changing nature of human experience and the role of choice and meaning in determining human action (Polkinghorne, 1983).

In working with people who have health problems, nurses are constantly reminded of the reality that mind and body are a unity. Any one experience reflects and will be reflected in the whole. Individuals with whom nurses interact are not only cells, body organs, or minds, but people with all of these dynamic traits who have families and cultures, past histories, and futures. All people have personal values and beliefs that have undeniable influence on experiences of health and illness.

Nurses also recognize the unrealistic split between theory and practice. Nurse scholars, educators, and practitioners have urged the building of bridges between what we know and what we do in practice (Benner and Wrubel, 1989). Theory that has practice value will not emerge exclusively from the methods of science. Theory that draws on multiple patterns of knowing will provide a valuable link between the worlds of practice and theory so they are not perceived as separate.

We believe that a hierarchic distinction between ways of knowing is not useful as an approach to developing nursing knowledge. Not only does this view place science in a superior position to other forms of knowing, but it overlooks forms of knowing that are valuable and necessary, even though different in form from science. In this text we view knowing, knowledge, and the development of knowledge from a holistic perspective, in that no single form of knowledge or way of knowing is judged to be superior or inferior to any other form. Different ways of knowing are not judged against one another. Rather, different ways of knowing and of creating knowledge are each, in their own right, useful for some purpose. Science is well suited for some purposes but not for others. Nurses routinely encounter situations that require decisions and actions for which there are no "scientific" answers. In many of these situations, other forms of knowing provide insight and understanding. For example, ethical problems require methods that are suitable for addressing human values of "rights" and "responsibilities."

Carper (1978) examined nursing literature and described four patterns of knowing that nurses have valued and used in practice: (1) ethics, the component of moral knowledge in nursing; (2) esthetics, the art of nursing; (3) personal knowledge in nursing; and (4) empirics, the science of nursing. Each of the patterns of knowing described by Carper is equally necessary, with each pattern contributing an essential component for the practice of nursing. Taken together, the patterns provide a basis for developing comprehensive knowledge. The following sections of this chapter present a conceptualization of how knowledge can be developed in nursing by drawing on Carper's four patterns of knowing.

THE WHOLE OF KNOWING

Nursing's patterns of knowing are interrelated processes that arise from the whole of experience. Informal, common, or everyday forms of knowing, as well as more formal ways of developing knowledge, contribute to useful knowledge for a practice discipline. In this text we use the term "knowing" to refer to the individual human processes of experiencing and comprehending the self and the world in ways that can be brought to some level of conscious awareness. Knowing is a dynamic, changing process. We use the term "knowledge" to refer to knowing that can be shared or communicated with others. Some forms in which knowledge is communicated are words, other symbols, actions, art, or sounds. Once expressed, knowledge can be passed along to others and can enter another person's conscious awareness.

Each of the patterns of knowing is a distinct aspect of the whole. Every pattern makes a unique contribution to the whole of knowing, and each is equally vital. Each pattern describes something about the whole of nursing knowledge. This construction of knowing provides a way to think about the purpose, expression, and processes for development of knowledge in nursing. However, the patterns "exist" only as dimensions of the whole of knowing in nursing and cannot be used separately from the whole. For example, an ethical problem in practice might be addressed at the outset using methods of dialogue and justification. As the situation unfolds in practice, aspects of empirics, personal knowing, and esthetics will also find expression, usually in synchrony with one another. The academic exercise of separating one pattern or another serves the purpose of refining ways of thinking and methods that contribute to an integrated process.

Fig. 1-1 is a representation of the whole of knowing based on each of the patterns originally described by Carper. In the figure, each shaded area represents a distinct pattern—ethics, esthetics, personal, and empirics—within the whole of knowing. Considering each pattern of the whole is like viewing a portion of the sky with a telescope; the telescope enlarges and brings into focus a distinct portion of the universe, but the viewer can also step away from the telescope and perceive the whole sky. Perception of each portion is influenced by the perception of the whole, and perception of the whole is also influenced by the ability to perceive each portion more clearly through the telescope.

Some form of expression is needed for each pattern so that what is created can be communicated and human methods for developing knowledge can proceed (Jacobs-Kramer and Chinn, 1988). As nurses practice, they know more than they can communicate. Some of what is "known" in practice can be expressed in words, actions, movements, or sounds, but much of what is "known" cannot be fully expressed. Attempting to express knowl-

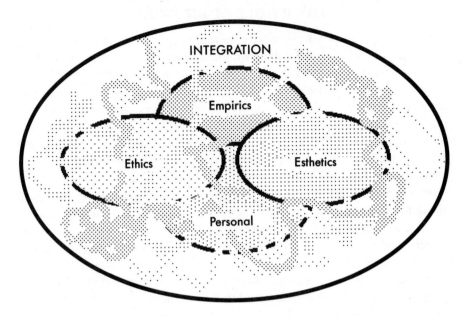

FIG. 1-1
The whole of knowing.

edge helps nurses focus, shape, influence, and communicate what is experienced. Expression makes it possible to move into a community, beyond the isolation of individual experience. Once this begins to happen, social purposes can form, and knowledge that helps the group to achieve their purposes can be shared. The process of developing shared knowledge opens possibilities for choices in nursing practice. The whole of knowing makes it possible to perceive what is possible and to create alternatives on which conscious choices can be made.

In Table 1-1 the creative and expressive dimensions of each pattern are described. The creative dimensions involve drawing on experience and "making sense" of that experience to move toward what can be or might be in the future. The expressive dimensions involve human actions—words, behaviors, and other symbols—that give communicable form to what we know and are not the same as what is "known." The creative dimensions are human activities that individuals can pursue alone or in which they can work in concert with others who share a common interest. Creative activities or processes are required to form the expressions that convey to others that which is understood or known. Two of the patterns of knowing, ethics and empirics, are expressed in familiar forms of language. The expression of the

TABLE 1-1
Patterns of knowing: creative and expressive dimensions

Dimension	Empirics	Ethics	Personal	Esthetics
Creative	Describing	Valuing	Opening	Engaging
	↕	↕	↕	↕
	Explaining	Clarifying	Centering	Interpreting
	↕	↕	↕	↕
	Predicting	Advocating	Realizing	Envisioning
Expressive	Facts, models, theories, descriptions	Ethical theory, principles, and guidelines	Authentic genuine self	Art/Act

patterns of esthetics and personal knowing is human actions and behavior rather than words. These human actions are also familiar, but they are commonly seen as expressions of personality or "art," not as expressions of human knowing or knowledge (Jacobs-Kramer and Chinn, 1988).

The traditions of science rest on the assumption that knowledge exists only to the extent that it can be objectified. Linguistic and mathematic forms of expression are the ideal in the scientific tradition. But, as the limits of empirics have become increasingly evident, it has become apparent that not all knowing can be communicated in language and, in fact, that language may distort the richness of human experience. Some form of communication is required for mutual understanding among people, but, because of its highly abstract nature, language also confounds shared understanding. As valuable and necessary as language is, it is not the only form of communication or expression that is available for human interaction. As other forms of expression come to be recognized and valued for their contribution to knowing processes, knowledge will become more whole and complete.

Empirics: the science of nursing

Empirics as the science of nursing emerged as a concept in nursing during the late 1950s (Carper, 1978). Empirics as a pattern of knowing draws on traditional ideas of science in which reality is viewed as something that can be verified by other observers. Empirics is based on the assumption that what is known is that which is accessible through the senses—that which can be seen, touched, heard, and so forth. The development of empiric knowledge has traditionally been accomplished by the methods of scientific hypothesis testing. Although most conceptualizations of empiric knowledge in nursing are linked to this traditional view of science, ideas about what is legitimate for the science of nursing have broadened to include activities that are not strictly within the realm of hypothesis testing such as phenomenologic descriptions or inductive (grounded) means of generating theory.

The processes related to creating empiric knowledge are describing, explaining, and predicting (see Table 1-1). A discipline focuses on a specific area of inquiry to describe, explain, and predict those things that are central to its purpose. Observations based on experience, facts, and impressions are expressed as organized descriptions. Empiric knowing may also be organized into conceptual models and theories that explain and predict relationships. These formally constructed ideas form what is commonly identified as a "body of knowledge."

Many of nursing's theories, conceptual models, and research efforts reflect an "ideal" of scientific inquiry. Nursing theories have been judged against the ideals of scientific theory. However, many traits of theories in general and nursing theories in particular both draw on and reflect other patterns of knowing besides empirics.

The ideal of scientific theory requires that all the major ideas of a theory be expressed in terms that can be "translated" to "out there" empiric reality. According to this ideal, if a theory addresses an idea of health, definitions of health should point to the specific behavior or traits that can be measured or at least inferred as representative of health. If one of these traits is blood pressure, the theory suggests which blood pressure values should be present to represent health. Nursing theorists have included specific observable traits and behaviors related to their ideas of health, but their writings also reflect the influence of individual values and beliefs regarding ideas such as health. Nursing theorists have also addressed the person of the nurse and the people with whom nurses interact, as well as insights that arise from the art of nursing. These dimensions of experience cannot be reduced to specific and measurable traits; thus patterns of knowing other than empirics are intrinsic to existing theories of nursing. As a result, when theories of nursing are judged against traditional ideals of science, they are thought to be lacking. When these same theories are viewed from the perspective of the whole of knowing, they assume a significance that moves beyond the limits of traditional science. In this text we focus on the development of theory that expresses empiric knowing.

Ethics: moral knowledge in nursing

Ethics in nursing is focused on matters of obligation or what ought to be done. The moral component of knowing in nursing goes beyond mere knowledge of the norms or ethical codes of nursing, other related disciplines, and society; it involves making moment-to-moment judgments about what should be done, what is "good" and "right," and what is "responsible." Making ethical judgments often involves confronting conflicting values, norms, interests, or principles. There may be no satisfactory answer to an ethical dilemma—only imperfect alternatives that require acting on the "lesser of two or more evils." Ethical knowing in nursing requires both an implicit knowing upon which difficult "on the spot" decisions are based, as well as knowledge of the formal principles and ethical theories of the discipline and society (Carper, 1978).

Creative processes of ethical knowing in nursing are clarifying, valuing, and advocating. The processes of valuing and clarifying explicate different philosophic positions about what is good, what is right, whose interest is being served, and which actions are responsible and the goals of those actions. Clarifying and valuing form the foundation for a personal ethic. These processes are used when nurses serve as advocates for the rights and responsibilities of others, as well as themselves.

Ethical knowledge is expressed in ethical theory, ethical principles, and ethical guidelines. It concerns the philosophic ideas upon which ethical decisions rest. Ethical knowledge does not describe or prescribe what a decision "should" be; rather, it provides insight as to what decisions are possible and why. Ethical theories are like empiric theories in that they can describe some dimensions of reality and can express relationships between phenomena. However, empiric theory relies on explicit reference to observable reality to be tested. Ethical theory cannot be "tested" in this sense because the relationships of the theory rest on underlying philosophic reasoning that cannot be empirically known. Empiric research can provide information and facts to guide the development of ethical knowledge and to assist in forming sound ethical decisions. However, empiric methods cannot be used to "test" ethical theory.

Personal knowing in nursing

Personal knowing in nursing concerns the inner experience of becoming a whole, aware self. As Carper states, "One does not know about the self, one strives simply to know the self." (Carper, 1978, p. 18). It is through knowing the self that one is able to know another human being as a person. Full awareness of the self, the moment, and the context of interaction makes possible meaningful, shared human experience. Without this component of knowing, the idea of "therapeutic use of self" in nursing would not be possible (Carper, 1978).

The creative processes of personal knowing are opening, centering, and realizing. Opening involves taking in the fullness of experience with conscious awareness. Centering is the process of contemplation and introspection that forms inner personal meaning from life experiences. Realizing is a process of expressing through personality, behavior, words, and deeds the genuine, real, whole self that is consistent with what is experienced in the inner life.

Unlike empirics and ethics, personal knowing is not directly communicable in language. The self is only fully communicated or described as the existence of self. What is perceived by others *is* the existence of the person or personality—the self. As personal knowing emerges more fully throughout life, the unique or genuine self can be more fully expressed and becomes accessible as a means by which deliberate action and interaction takes form. Although personal knowledge is not directly communicable in words, it is possible to describe certain things about the self. Self description is important in developing a shared understanding of how personal knowledge can be developed and used in a deliberative way. Descriptions about the self are limited in that they never fully reflect personal knowing, and they are retrospective in that they can only describe the self that was. However, descriptions can be a tool for developing self-awareness and self-intimacy and for communicating to others valuable ways of developing personal knowing (Hagan, 1990).

Esthetics: the art of nursing

Esthetic knowing in nursing is the comprehension of meaning in a singular, particular, subjective expression that we call the art/act. Esthetic knowing makes it possible to move beyond the limits and circumstances of a particular moment, to sense the meaning of the moment, and to envision what is possible but not yet real. Esthetic knowing in nursing is made visible through the actions, bearing, conduct, attitudes, and interactions of the nurse in response to others. Esthetic knowing is what makes possible knowing what to do with the moment, instantly, without conscious deliberation. The esthetic pattern of knowing makes possible the transformation of the immediate encounter into a direct perception of what is significant in it— that is, knowing or imparting meaning to what is being expressed in the encounter. Perception of meaning in an immediate encounter is what creates an artful nursing action, and the nurse's perception of meaning is reflected in the action taken (Carper, 1978).

Esthetic knowing involves the creative processes of engaging, interpreting, and envisioning. Engaging is a direct involvement of the self within a situation. The experience does not depend on mental structures or cognitive representations or explanations. Rather, the meaning of the moment comes from deep within the subjective experience, is interpreted from the context of the individual's human experiences and becomes expressed through in-the-moment being in the situation. Interpretation makes possible creative responses to the unique meaning of the moment and envisioning of new creative possibilities. As esthetic knowing develops, the art/act of nursing emerges; that is, the nurse's actions take on the element of artistry, creating unique, meaningful, deeply moving interactions with others that touch common chords of human experience.

Like personal knowing, esthetics is not expressed in language but artistically in the moment of experience-action. We refer in this text to the expression of the art/act, because nursing's art form tends to be the artful ways in which nurses interact with people and perform skilled tasks (Benner, 1984; Benner and Wrubel, 1989). The possibility for using the mediums of cultural art forms such as music, dance, and poetry also exist and are beginning to be explored in nursing (Watson, 1988).

Each art/act is a unique and particular instance that cannot be replicated; the creation of each art/act exists only in the moment. What is expressed as a work of art, an act, arises from and comprises the esthetic experience. As with personal knowing, knowledge about the processes and experiences of esthetics can be communicated retrospectively, and components of skills involved in esthetic knowing can be shared. For example, active listening is a component of empathic behavior that can be associated with esthetic knowing in nursing. Certain traits of active listening can be communicated, and the behaviors associated with active listening can be learned. However, esthetic knowing is expressed directly in the art/act; it only occurs in the moment and is unique to the particular esthetic experience. What is shared in the art/act becomes part of shared understanding in the form of esthetic knowledge, allowing for appreciation of the experience of the other.

PROCESSES FOR FORMING UNDERSTANDING

Nursing's patterns of knowing provide ways for sharing insights and understanding that can be used in practice. By understanding, we mean integrated comprehension that includes taking in the significance, background meanings, facts, and experiences as a whole. Understanding implies taking a perspective regarding "truth" that is open and dynamic; understanding does not imply utter certainty. Understanding includes what is "known" in a personal sense and in a collective sense as "knowledge." It also implies bringing a critical perspective to that which is known in order to create new insights and new knowledge. Each pattern of knowing has its own unique, distinct method for forming understanding. These methods are directly influenced

TABLE 1-2

Patterns of knowing: processes for forming understanding

Processes	Empirics	Ethics	Personal	Esthetics
Critical question	What is this? How does it work?	Is this right? For whom? Is this responsible?	Do I know what I do? Do I do what I know?	What does this mean?
Social/political process	Replication ↕ Validation	Dialogue ↕ Justification	Response ↕ Reflection	Consensus ↕ Criticism

by the creative and expressive dimensions of each of the patterns, but they also provide bridges for integrating the whole of knowing that is more than the sum of the parts.

Table 1-2 summarizes the processes for forming understanding. The processes for each pattern include critical questions that are addressed and social/political processes of interaction. The "social/political process" is comprised of interactive methods that are carried out in relation to the expression of each pattern of knowing. These methods reflect traditions and philosophic foundations on which the pattern of knowing rests. The methods represent a form of human interaction whereby the individual and the group find a common ground for making sense of the world. We have called these methods and interactions a "social/political process" to convey that forming understanding depends on the totality of culturally acquired expectations for human interactions, the influence of the particular period of history, the trends of the time, the place, and the social order. The process of forming understanding begins with fundamental critical questions that reflect the nature of each pattern of knowing. The questions that we suggest here are not the only questions that might be posed, but are representative of the basic questions that tend to direct the activities of inquiry arising from that pattern. Each method has its own style, its own variety and types of approaches, and its own perspective for judging the adequacy of the method itself. The methods growing out of the social/political process make it possible to integrate each of the patterns of knowing into a whole. Once the processes for forming understanding are engaged, regardless of the starting pattern, the processes of integration make all patterns accessible and create movement between and among the processes for the other patterns of knowing.

Replication and validation are the processes of empirics that contribute to understanding. Because of the familiarity of these processes in traditional science, replication and validation are sometimes mistakenly assumed to be appropriate as methods for other patterns of knowing. However, replication and validation are only useful for empirics. These processes require systematic empiric investigation that addresses such fundamental questions as: "What is this?" "How does it work?" Replication and validation require consistent agreement between people; what is thought to be for one person or context must hold "true" for another. For example, any one test that produces evidence related to a scientific theory is expected to be replicable in another time and situation to determine if the realities still hold true even with changing circumstances.

The social/political process of the ethical pattern of knowing is dialogue and justification. Critical questions that are addressed in relation to this pattern of knowing include: "Is this right?" "For whom?" "Is this responsible?" Ethical knowing does not require agreement in order to form understanding. Rather, ethical justification requires that fundamental value assumptions are made explicit and a line of reasoning emerges so that others can follow the basis upon which the individual reaches an ethical conclusion (theory, principles, guidelines). As ethical knowledge is expressed, dialogue becomes the social/political process so that the ideas are challenged, rethought, re-formed, and made clearer. This process makes it possible for a group to examine carefully the ethical basis for actions with respect to the group's collective and agreed-upon purposes or intents.

Reflection and response are the methods of personal knowing that contribute to understanding. The critical question that is addressed is: "Do I know what I do and do I do what I know?" Reflection requires the integration of a wide range of information and understanding derived from all forms of knowing and from other knowers, and an internal accounting of how fully that which is known is actualized or realized within the self of the knower. Responses from others mirror or "reflect back" the ways in which the person is perceived. As the responses of others are received, the individual gains insights that can be used in the self-reflection process, and the self becomes, or is realized, as an authentic being in the world.

Criticism and consensus are the social/political processes that contribute to forming understanding in esthetics. The critical question that is asked in relation to this pattern of knowing is: "What does this mean?" Criticism is a method that reveals meanings; it focuses on creating insights that can move beyond "what is" to something that "might be" in the future. Criticism is defined as "deliberate, critical, precise, thoughtful reflection and action directed toward transformation" (Wheeler and Chinn, 1989, p. 37).

The method of criticism as we envision it draws on criticism as used in the arts, where

> The art critic brings to the art insights and interpretations that help others to appreciate more fully what the artist has done, and what the art means for the culture as a whole. The critic does not proclaim the "correct" view of the art, but does provide a well-informed, knowledgeable interpretation of the art that helps others understand the art better, even if they don't agree with the views of the critic (Wheeler and Chinn, 1989, p. 37).

Rather than seeking agreement, esthetics depends on the process of consensus, where individuals bring to full awareness the diverse perspectives of others in the group, comprehending the realities of those perspectives, and integrating knowledge of those perspectives. Consensus depends on an "empathic move" that places each individual in the situation of the other, so that the perspective of the other can be fully appreciated. Out of this grows the capacity for the artful, deeply human interactions that are central to nursing practice.

INTEGRATION

Although the methods of each pattern of knowing can be described as distinct, each of the methods for forming understanding leads to integration of all patterns of knowing. The complete process of forming understanding provides a means for making explicit those insights that can be brought to awareness with respect to the whole of knowing. For example, the processes of empiric replication and validation involve artistic creativity, ethical choices, and personal perspectives. When all of the elements of knowing come together to form a whole, human understanding shifts toward possibilities that are greater than the sum of the parts. The method of one pattern cannot be used in relation to another pattern. However, as integration emerges with full consciousness, the methods of all of the patterns can come together.

As Carper demonstrated in identifying the patterns of knowing, nursing has a long history of drawing on or using various patterns. What has been missing is an explicit recognition of the value of all patterns of knowing as legitimate sources of knowledge for collective nursing knowledge.

Ethical knowing has been recognized as necessary in an increasingly crowded, complex technologic society, but the empirically discernible factors that are associated with ethics have been valued above the philosophic methods that are needed to create new ethical knowledge in nursing. Likewise, personal knowing has been acknowledged as an important component of nursing practice in order to develop the type of interpersonal relationships that are recognized as "therapeutic." However, personal knowing has not been viewed as a legitimate or formal source of new knowledge. Like personal knowing, esthetics has been recognized as an important source of insight for nursing practice; but esthetics has not been explored or valued as a potential source for the development of new knowledge. Both personal knowing and esthetics have been kept private, with little attention given to developing forms for their expression. Each pattern of knowing is distinct in its expression and its methods for contributing to understanding. Each pattern is equally necessary for full understanding, full knowing, the development of a collective body of knowledge, and nursing practice (Carper, 1978).

PATTERNS GONE WILD

When knowledge within any one pattern is not critically examined and integrated with the whole of knowing, distortion instead of understanding is produced. Failure to integrate all of the patterns of knowing leads to uncritical acceptance, narrow interpretation, and partial utilization. We call this "the patterns gone wild." When this occurs, the patterns are used in isolation from one another, and the potential for integration is lost.

Empirics removed from the context of the whole of knowing produces control and manipulation. Ironically these have been explicit traditional goals of the empiric sciences. When the validity of empiric knowledge is not questioned, it is used in contexts in which it does not belong. Once the value of all patterns of knowing are recognized, the goals of control and manipulation become evident as a distortion or misuse of empiric knowledge.

Ethics removed from the context of the whole of knowing produces rigid doctrine and insensitivity to the rights of others.

Personal knowing removed from the context of the whole of knowing produces isolation and self distortion. When this happens, the self remains isolated, and knowledge of self comes only from what is known internally. Self distortions can take a wide range of forms, from aggrandizement and overestimation of self to destruction and underestimation of self.

Esthetics removed from the context of the whole of knowing produces prejudice, bigotry, and lack of appreciation for meaning. Human actions become self-serving, shallow, arrogant, and empty. Human actions that reflect social prejudice and bigotry also grow out of a failure to comprehend the reality of the other, an assignment of unauthentic meanings to another's behavior, or assuming a self-serving posture with respect to another person.

To illustrate the "patterns gone wild," imagine an elderly woman admitted to a nursing home. She has lived a life rich in experience and activities and loves to verbally explore her past, making sense of what it means and how it relates to her present life. Having always been physically active, it is her practice to take a nightly stroll before going to bed. In the nursing home, she climbs over the bedrails after "lights out" and, with her walker, walks the halls, unsteady but determined, smiling and peering into other rooms. Sometimes, hearing another resident talking or moaning, she goes into the room and tells them stories or talks with them to ease their troubled night.

Consider what you might see in a nursing care plan if any one of the patterns of knowing were isolated from the context of the whole of knowing. "Empirics" might find and give a drug that would be effective in bringing sleep to the woman soon after the lights go out, thereby controlling the situation and manipulating her into compliance, regardless of any other concerns. "Ethics" might pass a rule that would punish the woman if she left her bed after the lights went out, creating a rigid, rule-oriented atmosphere that is insensitive to the rights of the woman and others. "Personal knowing" would not see the opportunity to reflect the meaning of the woman's experience within the self, but might simply grumble that the old woman is a nuisance and trouble, interfering with the time needed to complete the charting for the night. "Esthetics" might strap the woman to her bed, based on the prejudiced idea that this experience has no meaning, that old people are too frail and feeble to wander around the halls, and that by doing so they might hurt themselves.

When ethical, esthetic, and personal knowing, as well as empirics are integrated, the purposes of developing knowledge and the actions based on that knowledge become more responsible and humane, thus creating choice.

CONCLUSION

In this chapter we considered nursing's patterns of knowing and introduced ideas about how the whole of knowing emerges. We have described traits of each pattern—empiric, ethical, esthetic, and personal knowing. We introduced ideas about creative processes and forms of expressing knowledge that emerge from each of the patterns of knowing. There are methods suited to each pattern that can contribute to the process of forming understanding. The methods of personal knowing, ethics, and esthetics are introduced here and will be further developed in another text. In Chapter 2, we consider theory as an expression of empirics, which forms the focus for this book.

Nursing's patterns of knowing

REFERENCES

Benner P: From novice to expert: excellence and power in clinical nursing practice, Menlo Park, 1984, Addison-Wesley.

Benner P and Wrubel J: The primacy of caring, Menlo Park, 1989, Addision-Wesley.

Bleich D: Subjective criticism, Baltimore, 1978, Johns Hopkins University Press.

Carper BA: Fundamental patterns of knowing in nursing, Adv Nurs Sci 1(1):13–23, 1978.

Chinn PL: Debunking myths in nursing theory and research, Image, 17(2):45–49, 1985.

Hagan KL: Internal affairs: a journalkeeping workbook for self-intimacy, New York, 1990, Harper & Row.

Jacobs-Kramer MK and Chinn PL: Perspectives on knowing: a model of nursing knowledge, Scholarly Inquiry Nurs Pract 2(2):129–139, 1988.

Kerlinger FN: Foundations of behavioral research, ed 3, New York, 1986, Holt, Rinehart & Winston, Inc.

Polkinghorne D: Methodology for the human sciences, Albany, 1983, SUNY Press.

Watson J: New dimensions of human caring theory, Nurs Sci Q 1(4):175–181, 1988.

Wheeler CE and Chinn PL: Peace and power: a handbook of feminist process, ed 2, New York, 1989, National league for nursing.

2

Nursing theory as an expression of empirics

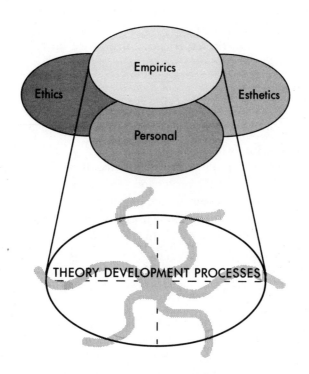

Empiric theory is one expression of empirics. Empiric theory contributes to nursing's identity, coherence of purpose, and ability to communicate within nursing and with people in related professions. Four processes integrate to create empiric theory. These are influenced by nursing's heritage and values and resources that evolve from the past.

In this book we primarily focus on understanding, developing, and examining one form of empirics, i.e., the range of theory that expresses empiric knowledge. Our discussion of empiric theory draws on generally accepted ideas about scientific theory and what it is, as well as our own ideas of empiric theory as a human science and a practice profession. Theorizing is often thought of as a cognitive or mental phenomenon, but, in our view, theory is developed by being and acting in the world. We also believe that reasoning and logic and the experiences of practice must be integrated to express the most useful empiric knowledge.

WHAT IS THEORY?

Defining "theory" can be complex, and ultimately most people accept an arbitrary meaning. Just when a definition seems firm, another idea surfaces that must be integrated into it. Like most terms, theory has many meanings, both within and outside of the profession of nursing. Theory has common, everyday connotations apparent in such phrases as . . . "I have a *theory* about that" or . . . "my *theory* is . . . ." These usages imply that theory is an idea or feeling or that it explains something. In this book we have used a definition that is consistent with these everyday meanings of theory as a collection of ideas or explanatory hunches. But our definition goes beyond this to a characterization of theory as something deliberately designed and created for a specific purpose.

In the broad, generic sense we have defined empiric theory as a systematic abstraction of reality that serves some purpose.

Systematic abstraction suggests both that there is an organized pattern underlying the creation and design of theory, as well as the idea that theory is not reality itself. For example, a mosaic is an art form that represents a type of systematic abstraction. A mosaic does not evolve from haphazardly adding individual tiles to a background. It is created when the designer carefully plans how the tiles should be arranged to form a pattern. The form to be achieved, which exists in the artist's mind, represents an idea or constellation of ideas. Like the mosaic, theory has organization and pattern. The organization of abstract ideas occurs with the use of disciplined, systematic thought and action.

Our broad definition of theory also implies that what is systematized is abstract. It is a representation of reality, not reality itself. The words and other symbols within theory are labels that stand for perceptual experiences of objects, properties, or events. For example, the word "book" is a word or label for an object you are presently reading. The word is not the object it represents. To illustrate the difference, close your eyes and conjure up an image of a book. To imagine a book without actually touching or seeing it is a relatively easy task if you have a mental image of what a book is like. You can imagine a "book" because the word "book" stimulates a mental image or abstraction that represents the object. Theory is made up of words (the label or word "book") that represent abstractions (mental image "book") of empiric experiences (object "book"). The words or symbols that express theory allow those theories to be communicated and understood.

In summary, theory as a systematic abstraction of reality implies an organization of words (or other symbols) that represent perceptual experiences of objects, properties, or events. Because there are many processes by which these abstractions are systematized, theory takes many forms. But the process is always systematic, and the form is always patterned.

Although theory is a systematic abstraction of reality, including nursing reality, it is also purpose oriented. Just as the processes used in designing theory may vary, the purposes for creating theory will vary. The creative dimensions of empiric theory are description, explanation, and prediction. Description means that abstractions of reality are systematized to account for something—to set forth what it is. Explanation implies that theory interrelates things to account for how they function. A theory can also predict under what conditions something will occur. These purposes of theory are fundamentally different, yet interrelated. To illustrate, think of "pain" as a central theoretic idea. It is quite a different task to describe pain, to explain how pain occurs, or to predict its occurrence. It is quite possible to predict pain without being able to explain or describe mental and physical processes that determine its manifestations. Descriptions of pain experiences can be extremely useful to nurses and may help nurses account for or predict pain in the absence of explanatory and predictive theory.

WHY DOES NURSING NEED THEORY?

One answer to the question "why theory in nursing?" is that theory can contribute to a well-founded basis for practice. A common response to questions about the value of theory is to point to past and present problems in nursing that might be solved through theory development or at least partially understood in relation to the presence or absence of theory. For example, many nursing procedures have been taught and practiced simply because they have always been done that way. If a theoretic rationale exists for changing practice, the alternative can be considered in light of this rationale, and an informed choice can be made about implementing it.

One recurrent myth about theory comes from the tendency to separate the "theoretic" from the "practical," thus creating the idea that theory is useless. This myth may be reinforced when broad nursing theories are examined, particularly by a practitioner seeking specific guidelines to assist in practical decisions about nursing care, because some of the practice implications in the broad theories are not direct or immediately obvious. Formulations that are commonly recognized as nursing theories represent the nursing world as it ought to be or might be, which is different from the nursing world in which practitioners function. As theorists and practitioners work together to understand and develop theories, this gap will become increasingly smaller. When a nursing theory is not sufficiently useful, one approach is to revise the theory. Another approach is to examine the issues about practice that the theory raises. Once practice is viewed in light of the theory, the theory gains a dimension of usefulness for changing practice.

Addressing the question, "Why is theory useful?" can enable both practitioners and theorists to form better relationships between their two worlds. The mere existence of theory provides a sounding board for basic assumptions and values about nurses and nursing and the ultimate purposes for which nursing practice exists. If a theory seems to lead practice in a direction that is inconsistent with the fundamental caring values of nursing practice, that theory might be rejected, regardless of how well it can be applied in practice. This has occurred in some instances in which nurses have seen Skinnerian behaviorist theory as leading to dehumanizing and uncaring practices in nursing.

Theory and professional identity

Theory is important for guiding nursing education, research, and practice and for strengthening the links between nurses who perfom these roles. How theory and identity are linked may be illustrated by considering the general area of family dynamics. Having theoretic knowledge develops an understanding of factors that affect family function. By basing their care on theoretic knowledge about family dynamics, nurses are able to work with families to help create healthy functioning. The effect of theory as a source of professional identity and unity is circular. As theoretic knowledge about family function is refined, nurses develop common understanding about nursing practice with families and base their practice on the theories that are useful. Practice, in turn, influences further development of the theories.

Professional identity that evolves out of theory provides a basis from which nurses can control the aspects of their practice. Nursing practice has traditionally been controlled by others, and what nurses do is often invisible. Hospital bills, for example, typically do not show nursing costs, leaving the impression that nurses provide no billable services. Theory that guides practice provides a language for talking about the nature of nursing practice and for demonstrating its effectiveness. Once nursing practice is described, it is made visible. When its effectiveness can be shown, it can be deliberately shaped or controlled by those who practice it.

On an individual level theory can provide a basis for self identity and esteem as a nurse. When you study theory and learn to make choices about its development and use, you will have a firmer base when your ideas are questioned. As you become familiar with the language and processes of theoretic knowledge development, you can begin to think about how assumptions, definitions, and relationships within theories can be challenged. The study and understanding of theory provides a basis upon which to take risks, to act deliberately, and to improve practice.

Imagine yourself as a nurse using hot, wet packs to ease chronic pain for a hospitalized person. A physician discovers that you are using this method of treatment, even though it isn't prescribed. Since this is an approach that is not familiar to the physician, she asks you about the packs. You explain your reasoning, which is based on theory. You also can provide research evidence of the method's effectiveness and information about the positive results that this particular person is experiencing. Your explanation leads to an informed discussion about various methods of pain management and why your approach seems to be effective for this person. As other practitioners learn of your knowledge in this area, they seek your consultation in pain management. Your knowledge of pain theory and what works in managing pain provides a valuable resource for developing and improving practice.

This incident is idealistic, but it does illustrate the potential of a theoretic foundation for professional identity. Theories, especially those developed in conjunction with practice, provide one avenue for developing both individual and collective identity.

Theory and coherence of purpose

The many varying points of view concerning the purpose of nursing are reflected in the following questions:
- Should nurses address prevention of illness?
- Should nurses treat human responses to illness?
- Should educational programs be structured around nursing process? Nursing diagnosis? Patterns of knowing?
- Should nurses view health and illness as opposites?
- Can ill people also be healthy?

Coherence of professional purpose is linked to professional identity. Coherence of purpose contributes to a collective identity when nurses agree on the general practice domain. Theory can help resolve significant disagreements among practitioners about what is to be accomplished.

For example, suppose a theory has been developed by and for nurses that directs practice toward health maintenance functions. This theory, in part, defines the parameters of health and is useful in guiding practitioners toward maintaining it. If nurses were to use this theory, health maintenance would emerge as a special expertise of nursing. The emergence of health maintenance as our unique role would be communicated within nursing, and the identity of professional nursing would be clearer.

Theory facilitates coherence by providing a basis for deliberate choices. Theory directs nursing toward some purpose other than "filling in a gap." When nurses agree about professional purposes and develop theory related to those purposes, the public and other practitioners will recognize nursing's expertise in relation to that theoretic arena. The fact that nurses are responsible for certain phenomena will be directly and indirectly communicated to society at large, and professional identity and coherence of purpose will evolve.

A somewhat simple and imprecise example may help to illustrate the value of theory in developing coherence of purpose. Suppose you wish to drive across the United States from the Pacific coast to the Atlantic coast. Both Maine and Florida are attractive and acceptable destinations, and the people going with you have mixed opinions about the relative merits of each. Your decision about where to go is the initial decision and quite separate from the choice of how to get there. Deciding on your destination will influence your decision about the route to take. But, on the other hand, your destination can depend on the options you perceive for getting there. If your group wishes to ride a train and the only train service is to Maine, you might decide on your destination and your route because you want to ride the train. If you decide to get in a car and just drive, with the purpose of experiencing whatever you find across the continent, you are likely to have a good trip, but you will not be able to assure anyone as to where you will be going.

This example illustrates some of the considerations that nurses might take into account in developing theory. Having a purpose, or a destination, is not essential, but it does help to shape complex decisions when many different people are involved. As coherent purposes for nursing emerge, the means of attaining the goals and the relative merits of journeying one way or another can be carefully considered.

Theory and professional communication

All theory, regardless of type, helps to enhance communication. The study of theory by practicing nurses and students of nursing provides a common foundation of knowledge and thought from which to practice. If knowledge of existing theory within nursing is essential, all students of nursing should be familiar with nursing's theoretic knowledge and understand the basics of theory development.

If theory is to be useful for practice, theorists must be concerned about how theory relates to the practice arena. We believe it is essential to communicate with the world of practice to foster professional communication.

Using the example of pain management, if a theorist were devising a theory to guide pain management for people with chronic pain, pain would be an idea (concept) of key importance within the theory. Since the word "pain" represents a complex abstraction, pain alleviation could mean many things. Suppose the theorist intends to develop the theory by using research to test the effectiveness of two or three pain alleviation methods. The theorist and researchers must determine how to empirically represent the pain phenomena. Some of the decisions that must be made are: (1) how to think about and assess pain, (2) how to relate the pain experience to the treatment, and (3) how to determine pain relief, which in turn would indicate treatment effectiveness.

One choice for assessing pain is to monitor neural response using a skin electrode attached to a laboratory instrument. When assessed this way, pain is "seen" as an oscilloscope display of frequency and amplitude of action potentials. The effectiveness of the tested nursing intervention is determined by alterations in the neural response that in turn represent pain.

A second choice for representing pain can be quite different. Rather than an oscilloscope tracing, a score derived from observing body movement and the person's report of the pain experience are used to assess pain. The difference between assessing pain from a neural response and assessing pain from observation of behavior illustrates how the word "pain" can legitimately be assessed in different ways, and either assessment approach is reasonable.

Suppose the research team chooses to assess the effectiveness of two different pain management methods by bringing people to the laboratory and monitoring their neural response using the oscilloscope tracing. When this clinically impractical method of assessing pain is chosen, it is difficult to transfer the ideas of the theory into practice. For one thing, variables that operate in the clinical area are not operating in the laboratory setting. Second, the nurses have no way of knowing how neural response patterns relate to the subjective experience of pain. If the research team chooses to use the subjective response scale to represent pain, the theory lends itself to further clinical testing, since the pain assessment technique considers the subjective pain response.

When a theory is developed using research, the choices about how to represent ideas (concepts)—in this example, pain—will determine how useful the theory is. A theory that is useful for practice enhances communication between theorists, researchers, and nurses in practice. If theory is to enhance professional communication, it must be developed in a way that maximizes its utility for practice.

Some theories do not initially and immediately address clinical nursing concerns. In fact, theory that is useful for practice can be rooted in research that is quite remote from nursing care environments. Ultimately, however, theory development should arise from some frame of reference that addresses nursing concerns in a way that enhances communication between nurses in practice and those developing the theory.

What kind of theory?

In recent nursing literature there are discussions about what constitutes *nursing* theory. Should nursing have theories *about* nursing? *For* nursing? Or *in* nursing? Is basic theory important? Is broad theory about health care systems important? The answer to these and related questions is—yes! We believe that many types of theory covering many areas are needed in nursing. However, to answer "yes" to all these questions does little to resolve the difficulty of knowing which choice to make between alternate approaches at any given time. In our opinion the choice should be guided by an explicit purpose or concern that can be communicated to others and is seen as reasonable or important by others in the discipline.

Theory in nursing contributes to communication among practitioners, to clarifying the purposes of nursing, and to forming professional identity. Theory is not the only "answer"; and, as with other professions, there are personal and political issues that affect its development. The processes and products of theory development help to transcend the personal and political problems, providing a substantive foundation from which to work.

HOW DOES A DISCIPLINE ACQUIRE THEORY?

There are four processes for creating empiric theory, which are shown as quadrants in Fig. 2-1. When all of these processes occur, theory with practical value evolves. Central to each of the processes is a historical core from which curved lines emanate. The wave lines represent current situations and circumstances that have roots in nursing history. The lines separating each

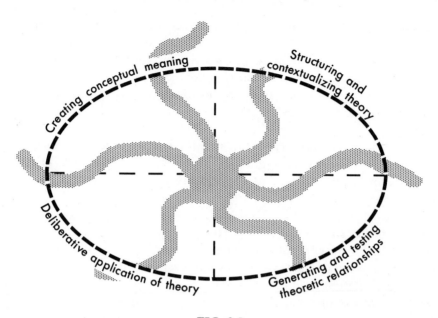

FIG. 2-1
A process for theory development.

quadrant illustrate that each process is different from, but continuous with, other processes. The processes are enclosed by broken lines to symbolize that there is open communication between nursing's theory development processes and similar processes in other professions and disciplines, but that boundaries still exist.

Processes for theory development

Each of four major processes contributes to the development of theory in a practice discipline (see Fig. 2-1). These are (1) creating conceptual meaning, (2) structuring and contextualizing theory, (3) generating and testing theoretic relationships, and (4) deliberative application of theory.

Creating conceptual meaning. This is the process of identifying, examining, and clarifying the mental images that comprise the elements, variables, or concepts within theory. This process is applied particularly to the major concepts around which a theory is developed.

Structuring and contextualizing theory. This is the process of organizing relationships between and among concepts in a rigorous and systematic way, consistent with the purposes of the theory. This process also includes identifying the domain, realm, or context of the theory, stating the assumptions upon which the theory is based, and providing conceptual definitions of terms that guide decisions about the empiric events to which concepts relate.

Generating and testing theoretic relationships. This process has three subcomponents: (1) empirically grounding emerging relationships, (2) explicating empiric indicators, and (3) validating the relationships through empiric methods.

Deliberative application of theory. This is the process of using research to evaluate the effectiveness of a theory in achieving the goals of nursing practice. Research can provide evidence of how useful theory is in practice.

A detailed explanation of each of these processes is found in Chapter 5. The remainder of this chapter focuses on the influence of history, resources, and values on theory development processes within nursing.

The heritage of history

We have depicted the heritage of nursing history by a circle in the center of Fig. 2-1. History influences the present direction of theory development. To a great extent, history determines nursing's area of concern. History changes in an accumulative manner; it can be added to but never subtracted from. The historical core has a boundary because, once history is made, it cannot be changed. Some historical factors influence current theory development more than others. These are shown as wave lines emanating from the historical core.

Wave lines

The wave lines from the inner core extend into each of the theory development processes and are curvilinear to convey the idea of change and movement. Since history changes as events evolve, its influence on theory changes.

The wave lines are circumstances that evolve from the past. There are two general types of circumstances—values and resources. Values and resources can be those of the individual, the professional group, or society. All wave lines extend beyond the open boundaries. This represents the idea that historically derived factors that influence the development of theory in nursing "reach out" to influence other groups with related theoretic concerns.

Quadrant lines

The horizontal and vertical lines represent the distinct nature of each process. The lines are not continuous because, even though each process influences and is influenced by the others, the processes are fundamentally different. The outcome of processes within one quadrant cannot be improved by improving the quality of processes within another quadrant. If, for example, the meaning you create for concepts is incomplete, the idea of the concept will not be improved by designing "better" theoretic relationships. If the meaning you create is incomplete, the relationships generated that depend on those meanings will also be inadequate. The conceptual meaning must be addressed first.

To illustrate the characteristics of the individuality yet mutual interrelatedness of each of the processes within the system, consider a family of four people. The family members are separate people; if you know one, you do not automatically know the others. Because the family members are mutually interdependent, you can infer characteristics of the group through knowledge of one member. If you know one member's dietary preferences, you have some clues as to what the nutritional patterns of the group might be, but you cannot empirically know until you ask each member or observe their behavior.

Each nurse who contributes to theory development will become more experienced and interested in using one or two of the theory development processes. To the extent that every nurse can appreciate the contributions made by all theory development processes, there will be more potential for development of useful theory in nursing.

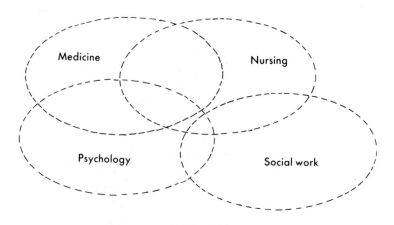

FIG. 2-2
Overlap of theory development processes among professions.

Theory and nursing: A systematic approach

Boundary lines

The boundary lines in Fig. 2-1 that enclose the theory development processes symbolize the idea that the domain of nursing is limited. But, even though the processes are bounded, there is free exchange of theoretic content and processes among different professions and disciplines. Fig. 2-2 illustrates how a group with different purposes can overlap theoretically. The labels we have chosen are arbitrary and are not meant to imply the degree or nature of overlap or separateness of the groups. The areas of overlap suggest that professions share areas of interest. The empiric domains of nursing and medicine overlap. Neither can realistically or effectively deal with all aspects of health and illness.

Both nursing and medicine are concerned, in part, with human experiences of health and illness. There is a wide range of health and illness experience; nursing and medicine each work with some common and some different aspects of these experiences. The differences are defined by the distinct purposes and aims of each group as a profession. Medicine aims to cure disease; nursing aims to alleviate the suffering that accompanies disease. Each of these aims is worthy; each concerns the human experience of disease. However, each of these aims is fundamentally different, requiring different types of knowledge and understanding.

USE OF THE PROCESSES FOR THEORY DEVELOPMENT

The processes for theory development are fluid, complex, and diverse. Together they form a unified whole. Individual nurses, with different talents and aptitudes, can contribute to the process of creating theory. Each individual typically develops skill with respect to one or two of the processes. Taken together, individual efforts form the whole of the field of inquiry.

Generally people have an inclination toward one or the other of these processes. If elusive abstract ideas are interesting to you, you may be impatient or bored with research processes required for testing or applying theory. If you prefer to deal directly with the clinical nursing world, you may be impatient with abstract ideas about practice. Your openness to and appreciation of the work of other nurses who use a mode different from yours is a key to creating a cohesive community within nursing. Ideally individuals with complementary talents and interests will form alliances or channels of communication and will deliberately assist one another. Literature that reflects diverse interests will facilitate understanding and cooperation. Researchers can benefit from philosophic and analytic work that focuses on the meanings of concepts. Theorists can use research reports as evidence that theories are empirically meaningful. Practitioners can use theory to create new approaches in practice. Each of the processes, operating in synchrony, can provide unity of purpose for nursing.

CONCLUSION

Empiric theory, the focus for this book, is one expression of empirics. Empiric theory contributes to the identity and coherence of purpose of nursing and to the ability to communicate within nursing and with people in related professions. There are four major processes that can be used to develop empiric theory. These processes are: creating conceptual meaning, structuring and contextualizing theory, generating and testing theoretic relationships, and deliberative application of theory. The processes are influenced by nursing historical heritage and the values and resources that evolve from the past.

3

Emergence of nursing theory

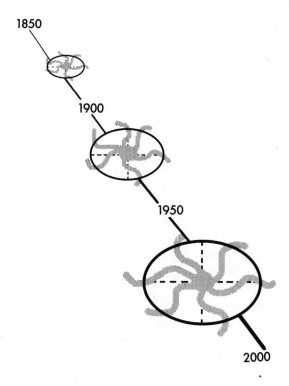

1850

1900

1950

2000

The values and resources influencing theory development are rooted in history. As early theorists developed a sense of community and scholarship, they influenced more recent theoretic developments. A perspective of history makes it possible to refine understanding of what theory is.

Current issues in nursing can be directly traced to the past and will continue to shape the future. Theory development draws directly on history and the circumstances that evolve from it. This chapter examines the history of nursing and the values and resources that affect theory development within the profession.

HISTORY OF THEORY DEVELOPMENT

Early in the development of nursing as a profession, leaders in nursing theorized about the nature of nursing practice, the principles on which practice is based, and the proper goals and functions of nursing in society. Early conceptualizations of nursing emphasized the art of nursing. By the 1950s nurses began to develop nursing science. Professional development and the development of nursing theory have a long and important history (Ashley, 1976).

Nightingale (1969, p.3), in establishing the discipline of nursing, spoke with firm conviction about the nature of nursing as a profession distinct from medicine. Nightingale conceived of nursing as a profession that could provide an avenue for young women to make a meaningful contribution to society.

In the mid 1800s women cared for the English sick as daughters, wives, mothers, or maids. This socially prescribed role influenced Nightingale's conviction that nursing should be a profession for women, but this cultural tradition was secondary to her philosophy. Her primary concern was the more pervasive plight of Victorian women. Women in her era were either poverty- stricken and forced to work at menial labor for long hours, or they were idle ornaments in the household of wealthy husbands or fathers. In either case, there was no avenue in which women could use their "intellect, passion, or and moral activity" to benefit society (Nightingale, 1980).

Nightingale spent the first decade of her adult life tormented by a desire to use her productive capacities in a way that would benefit society. She defied the wishes of her family and obtained formal training as a nurse and subsequently agreed to serve in the Crimean War (Nightingale, 1980; Tooley, 1905; Woodham-Smith, 1983). After her service in the war, Nightingale wrote *Notes on Nursing,* in which she set forth the basic premises on which nursing practice was to be based and articulated the proper functions of nursing. In her view, nursing functions included making astute observa-

34

tions of the sick and their environment, recording observations, and developing knowledge about the factors that promote the reparative process (Nightingale, 1969).

Firmly committed to the idea that nursing's responsibilities were distinct from those of medicine, Nightingale maintained that the knowledge developed and used by nursing must be distinct from medical knowledge. She insisted that early nursing schools should be controlled and staffed by women who were trained nurses. Trained nurses should also manage and control nursing practice in homes and hospitals. Nightingale influenced the establishment of schools of nursing in England and the United States. The first Nightingale schools were autonomous in their administration, and nurses held decision-making authority over nursing practice in institutions where students learned. Student learning in these schools emphasized the powers of observation, the necessity of recording observations, and the potential for organizing nursing knowledge gained through observation and recording. In addition, Nightingale held strong beliefs about the values that should be cultivated in nursing, and these values were reflected in the educational programs of early schools (Barnard and Neal, 1977; Dennis and Prescott, 1985).

After the Nightingale era many forces in society emerged in opposition to Nightingale's model. In the United States the medical care system developed as a capitalist, for-profit business. This system provided the context for rapid technologic development, as well as a complex industrial system to support medical interventions. Early in the 1900s, when the medical care system was taking shape as a science and as a political body, physicians and hospital administrators saw nurses as a source of inexpensive or free labor that could further their economic goals. Many women who entered nursing and who provided free student labor for hospitals were working-class women with limited opportunities for education. Nurses were exploited both as students and as trained, experienced workers and were viewed as submissive, obedient, and humble women who ideally fulfilled their responsibilities to physicians without question. Nurses' positive desire to help people in need, coupled with a relative lack of educational preparation and social or political power, led to an extended period in history when nursing was practiced primarily under the control and direction of medicine (Lovell, 1980).

Despite strong leaders who followed the Nightingale tradition and viewed nursing knowledge as unique, nursing's knowledge has not always been regarded as distinct from medicine. During the early 1900s most of the Nightingale-modeled schools in the United States were brought under the control of hospitals, and nursing education and practice were transferred from the profession to the control of hospital administrators and physicians

(Ashley, 1976). Consistent with the social history of women, nursing was viewed increasingly as a role supporting and supplementing medicine (Hughes, 1980; Lovell, 1980). Education for women and nurses was discouraged and limited. Women who were nurses were expected to follow orders and serve the needs and interests of physicians providing care (Melosh, 1982; Reverby, 1987). Economic independence for women was not possible until the mid 1900s. Even though a woman earned an income, she was not able to have a bank account, own property, or conduct financial transactions in her own name. Normal schools were established for the training of teachers, and nursing schools were available for training nurses, but to obtain long-term security, women were required to conform to the role of wife or daughter.

Throughout the early part of the twentieth century, nursing practice was based on rules, principles, and traditions that were passed along through limited apprenticeship forms of education. Further education was not available; thus much of what evolved as nursing knowledge was wisdom that came from years of experience. Principles for practice were sometimes derived from scientific knowledge. Many "principles" were generalizations from the theories of other disciplines such as Ohm's law related to pressure, resistance, and flow. Other principles came from generally accepted facts such as the fact that microbes could be transferred by means of object-to-object contact or by droplets in the air. Certain traditions of practice were thought to be sound but were never examined. For example, knowledge of the germ theory of disease and related propositions concerning the transmission of disease led to aseptic procedures in handling equipment, isolating individuals who were thought to be contagious, and hand-washing techniques. These approaches became traditions of practice because they were thought to be effective or "sound."

Tradition as a basis for nursing practice was perpetuated by the nature of apprenticeship education in nursing (Ashley, 1976). Student nurses were presumed to learn at random through long hours of experience, limited exposure to lectures or books, and accepting without question the prescriptions of practical techniques. The novice nurse acquired knowledge of what was "right" and "wrong" in practice by observing more experienced practitioners and by memorizing facts about the performance of nursing tasks. Nursing was viewed primarily as a nurturing and technical art requiring apprenticeship learning and innate personality traits congruous with the art (Ashley, 1976; Hughes, 1980).

Despite social impediments to the development of nursing knowledge, nursing philosophy and ideology remained committed to the idea that nursing requires a distinct body of knowledge for practice (Abdellah, 1969; Hall,

1964; Henderson, 1964, 1966; Rogers, 1970). This commitment grew from the consistently observed fact that, although the goals of nursing and medicine were similar and related, the central goals and functions of nursing required knowledge not provided by medicine or by any other single discipline outside of nursing.

Despite the social circumstances that limited nursing education, nursing leaders sustained ideals that reflected Nightingale's model. Because most nursing service was provided as free labor by students in hospitals, practicing graduate nurses functioned as independent practitioners engaged by families to assist in the care of the sick in homes and in hospitals. Nurse leaders became active in confronting a wide range of social and health issues of the time, including temperance, freedom for slaves, suffrage for blacks and women, and control of venereal disease.

There is substantial evidence that graduate nurses in the early part of the twentieth century contributed substantively to improving health conditions in hospitals, homes, and communities. They developed health knowledge and were politically active in finding ways to distribute this knowledge to people who needed it (Wheeler, 1985).

Consistently throughout the twentieth century, nursing leaders in the United States have called for social and political reforms to restore the control of nursing practice to nurses. Margaret Sanger, Lillian Wald, and Lavinia Dock are three nurses who led this effort early in the century. These nurses were challenged by specific needs of society and independently set about to develop their practice on the basis of what they saw as a need in health care. They observed the circumstances of people in their communities, identified a health-related need, and organized nurses to meet the needs. They recorded their observations and the conclusions that they drew from these observations. Sanger developed knowledge about reproduction and birth control. She fought against great odds to distribute birth control information to women who were desperate to obtain it and established a foundation for family planning programs that remains viable today (Sanger, 1971).

Wald became concerned about child care and family health in the context of extremely poor conditions of sanitation in the crowded immigrant tenements of New York City. She established the House on Henry Street in New York City from which she developed concepts of community health nursing and social welfare programs. She developed stations from which safe milk was distributed to families with young children and centers for educating mothers in the care of their families (Silverstein, 1985; Wald, 1971).

Dock was an ardent pacifist who worked with Wald at the Henry Street Settlement. While at Henry Street she campaigned actively for changes in labor laws that would benefit women and children. She devoted 20 years of her life to gain enfranchisement for women. Dock reasoned that if women could vote, the oppressive laws that affected them would be changed (Christy, 1969).

Lydia Hall is a more recent example of a nurse who constructed specific philosophic ideas about how nursing should be practiced and who implemented this philosophy in practice. She established Loeb Center at Montefiore Hospital in New York City. Loeb is a nursing center where nursing maintains control over the care provided and where people and their families have primary decision- making power over the kind of care that they receive (Hall, 1963).

Like theorists of today, these early nursing leaders developed and used knowledge as one means to bring about improvements in health care and nursing practice. Their work also reflected the conviction that nurses can and should control nursing practice, based on a strong knowledge base. Their work included making detailed observations, recording these observations, organizing the knowledge that came from their observations, and establishing guiding values and philosophies for practice.

Although many valuable traditions of nursing practice remain, the ideas of nursing as a science that began to take hold in the 1960s produced a significant change. Gradually nursing shifted from a fact-oriented perspective of what nursing is and what is "right" or "proper" in nursing practice to a questioning perspective that focuses more on what is effective nursing practice (Hardy, 1978).

The shift toward science as the basis for developing nursing knowledge was influenced by the involvement of nursing in the two world wars of the 1900s. The wars created social circumstances that brought about substantial shifts in roles for women and nurses. Many women were required to enter the skilled or unskilled labor force during the years when men were away in battle. During wars there were fewer home responsibilities, and women who were nurses were needed to support the war effort by providing care for the sick and wounded. War-related programs were instituted by the U.S. government to make training available to women who agreed to serve in the war (Kalisch and Kalisch, 1978; Kelly, 1985).

Partly because of the greater demand for skilled nurses to serve the war effort, by the decade of World War II women had begun to enter institutions of higher learning in greater numbers. Nursing leaders conceived of nursing education as being properly placed within colleges and universities. Early efforts to develop nursing research began in the context of the military, which provided support for nursing research. After the end of World War II, many educational programs were established within institutions of higher learning rather than in hospitals, and graduate programs for nurses began to appear. Academic institutions required faculty to hold advanced degrees and encouraged them to meet the standards of higher education with regard to service to community, teaching, research, and scholarship. Once nurses gained the skills to use the methods of science, nursing theories and other types of theoretic writings appeared.

In 1950 *Nursing Research,* the first nursing research journal, was established. Books on research methods and explicit theories of nursing began to appear. Early research reports are limited when compared to those of today, but these writings quickly changed and began to reflect qualities of serious scholarship and investigative skill. Various schools of thought emerged about the nature of nursing practice, providing a fresh flow of ideas that could be examined by members of the profession. These writings provided a stimulus for early efforts in developing theory.

By the 1960s doctoral programs in nursing were being established. With this development, committees of nurses began to formally consider the development of nursing knowledge. Nurse scholars began to debate ideas, points of view, and methods in the light of nursing's traditions (Hardy, 1978; Leininger 1976). These debates are reflected in the literature of the late 1960s and early 1970s (Dickoff and James, 1971; Dickoff, James, and Wiedenbach, 1968; Ellis, 1971; Folta,1971; Walker 1971, 1972; Wooldridge, 1971). Fundamental differences in viewpoints about nursing "science" provided nurse scholars the opportunity to learn, sharpen critical thinking skills, and acquire knowledge about the processes of science.

By the end of the 1970s, the number of doctorally prepared nurses in the United States had grown to nearly 2000. Approximately 20 doctoral programs in nursing had been established, and masters' programs were maturing in academic stature and quality. Masters' programs were focused on the preparation of advanced practitioners in nursing rather than on preparing educators and administrators. Three major trends that emerged during the 1960s and 1970s provided impetus for the development of nursing knowledge as a basis for nursing practice.

Conceptual models and philosophies of practice

First, nurses began to reconsider the nature of nursing and the purposes for which nursing exists. Nurses began to question the ideas that were taken for granted in nursing and the traditional basis on which nursing was practiced. They wrote and published their ideas about nursing and the type of knowledge, skills, and background needed for practice. Although many of the writings of the 1960s and 1970s were not intended as theories in a formal sense, they are significant contributions to the development of theoretic thinking in nursing. Many of these theoretic works have been used as a basis for curricula, and some have been applied in practice.

Many early nursing models and philosophies include a description of the nursing process. This process, which is similar to both the problem-solving and the research processes, is a framework for viewing nursing as a deliberate, reflective, critical, and self-correcting system. The nursing process replaced the rule- and principle-oriented approaches with a reflective problem- solving approach. The components of the nursing process were viewed as a basis for cultivating basic inquiry skills among nurses. Nursing diagnosis, which evolved from the nursing process, was seen as one means for organizing the domain of nursing practice. The early literature concerning nursing diagnosis included practical and theoretic ideas about developing a taxonomy of nursing diagnoses and testing their validity.

Conceptual models for nursing education and practice proliferated in the 1960s and 1970s. Philosophies of nursing science and nursing practice developed, with growing emphasis on esthetic, ethical, and personal components of nursing knowledge. As these ideas began to be used in practice settings, the relationships between nursing models and nursing practice have become clearer. Practicing nurses are finding a new sense of purpose and direction consistent with the basic values of nursing and a sense of the increasing effectiveness achieved through use of systematic and thoughtful forms of nursing practice. The ideas of Sister Callista Roy, Doretha Orem, Betty Neuman, and Imogene King are examples of theoretic ideas that have been applied in practice.

Theories borrowed from other disciplines

As the educational preparation of nurses expanded, theories that had been developed in other disciplines were recognized as important for nursing. Problems in nursing practice for which there had seemed no readily available solution began to be viewed as resolvable if theories from other disciplines were applied. For example, nurses recognized that young children needed the continuing love and support of their parents and families during hospitalization. The strict rules of hospitals that severely restricted visitation interrupted these primary family ties. As psychologic theories of attachment and separation developed, nurses found an explanation for the problems experienced by hospitalized children and were able to change visitation practices to provide sustained contact between parents and children.

Although theories from other disciplines have been useful in some instances, nurses have also exercised caution in arbitrarily applying these theories. In some instances the theories of other disciplines do not take into consideration significant factors that influence a nursing situation. For example, some theories of learning applicable to classroom learning do not adequately reflect the process of learning when an individual is faced with the stress of an illness. Although borrowed theories may be useful, their usefulness cannot be assumed until they are examined from the perspective of nursing in nursing situations (Whall, 1980).

The development of theory within the discipline

The early formal movement to develop theory originating from nursing was influenced by the writings of Dickoff and James and their colleagues. They described one view of how theory can be developed and the nature of theory for a practice discipline (Dickoff and James, 1968; Dickoff, James, and Wiedenbach, 1968). Their approaches were discussed in the literature and at conferences, reflecting a growing commitment of nurses to develop nursing theory. Although theories from other disciplines have been useful, they have not been sufficient to provide comprehensive understanding for nursing practice.

Some theories or models developed within nursing began as an effort to revise or extend theories in other disciplines. For example, Roy (1976) developed a model derived from the work of Helson, whose theory of adaptation was formulated to explain the function of the eye. Other theorists such as Dorothea Orem, Imogene King, and Virginia Henderson developed their ideas from observations of nursing practice and literature resources. Other approaches such as that of Rogers (1970) emerged out of a philosophic perspective about nursing and the nature of health and human experience.

MAJOR VIEWS EXPRESSED IN EARLY NURSING MODELS

From these developments in the history of nursing, philosophic foundations evolved that are now common elements in nursing theories and models. They include ideas about the nature of nursing, the nature of the person, society and environment, and health (Fawcett, 1978; Yura and Torres, 1975). The manner in which each of these ideas has been developed characterizes the nature of nursing as a distinct discipline and provides direction for the future development of nursing knowledge.

Nature of nursing

In nursing theory, nursing is generally represented as a helping process with a primary focus on interpersonal interactions between a nurse and another individual. This general idea does not clearly distinguish nursing from other helping disciplines, but it provides an important focus for deciding what kind of knowledge is needed in nursing practice. The interpersonal nature of nursing practice distinguishes nursing from medicine, in that medicine focuses on surgical and pharmacologic interventions, with interpersonal interactions as secondary to these interventions. For nursing, interpersonal interactions are primary, whereas technical and medical interventions support the primary interpersonal interactions.

Ideas in theoretic writings related to the nature of nursing are significant indicators of the esthetic component of nursing knowledge. For example, Ernestine Wiedenbach (1964) views nursing action taken in response to a person's need as a visible expression of the art of nursing. Hildegard Peplau (1952), Joyce Travelbee (1966, 1971), Josephine Paterson and Loretta Zderad (1976), and Patricia Benner (1984), have provided additional important contributions to conceptualizing the art of nursing.

Although different nurse authors present conceptualizations of the nature of nursing that are consistent with the idea of interpersonal interactions as a primary focus, there are important differences in their definitions and conceptualizations. For some authors, the direction of the interaction and the specific actions that are taken in achieving the goals of the interaction are largely defined by the person with whom the nurse interacts. The nurse's role in the interaction is primarily one of facilitating. When this view of the nature of nursing is incorporated into a theory or model, nursing is viewed as enabling the will and behavior of the person receiving care.

Other theories present a view of the interpersonal process as one that is either shared or initiated by the nurse. In this view, nursing processes and actions rest primarily on the nurse's initiative, knowledge, and approaches. The theoretic ideas that emerge from this view focus on nursing actions to reach the goal or purposes of the interaction.

Each of these perspectives is consistent with nursing, in that nurses encounter some situations in which the client primarily directs the interaction and others in which the nurse is the initiator. Some nursing theories account for this diversity. The common thread that is significant is the view of the primacy of human interaction in creating human health and wholeness. Table 3-1 describes the concept of nursing as reflected in the work of several nurse theorists.

The person

All nursing theories and models include ideas about the nature of human beings. The most consistent philosophic component of the idea of the person is the dimension of wholeness or holism. The nature of holism as a concept is difficult to address from the perspective of traditional Western philosophies based on the idea of reductionism. In the reductionist view of holism, the whole is equal to the sum of the parts; when interrelationships

TABLE 3-1

Theoretic ideas about nursing

Author	Concepts of nursing
Hildegard Peplau (1952)	Nursing is a significant therapeutic interpersonal process. The interpersonal process is a maturing force and educative instrument for both the nurse and the client. Self-knowledge in the context of the interpersonal interaction is essential to understanding the client and reaching resolution of the problem. There are four sequential phases of the interpersonal process: (1) orientation, (2) identification, (3) exploitation, and (4) resolution.
Ida Jean Orlando (1961)	Nursing is a process of interaction with an ill individual to meet an immediate need. The nursing situation consists of: (1) the person's behavior, (2) the nurse's reaction, and (3) nursing action appropriate to the person's need. The nurse is accountable to the individual receiving care.
Ernestine Wiedenbach (1964)	There are three components of nursing: (1) identification of a person's need for help, (2) ministration of the help needed, and (3) validation that the help provided was indeed helpful. The nursing process begins with an activating situation that arouses the nurse's consciousness. Clinical nursing has four components—philosophy, purpose, practice, and art.
Myra Levine (1967)	Nursing care is both supportive and therapeutic. Supportive interventions are designed to maintain a state of wholeness as consistently as possible with failing adaptation. Therapeutic interventions are designed to promote adaptation that contributes to health and restoration of health. All nursing actions are based on conservation of energy, structural integrity, personal integrity, and social integrity.

Theory and nursing: A systematic approach

among parts are understood, generalizations can be made about the whole (Newman, 1979). Western culture is based on this view, so that nurses, like others in this culture, have learned to think about parts of lives, parts of bodies, and parts of human experiences.

In a pure sense, holism means that the whole is greater than the sum of the parts and that the whole cannot be reduced to parts without losing something in the process. Some nursing theorists view the individual as a system of biologic, sociologic, and psychologic parts. This view is not consistent with holism in its purest sense, but there is still a strong commitment to the idea that all components of the individual need to be considered (Flaskerud and Halloran, 1980). Martha Rogers, Margaret Newman, Joyce Travelbee, and Patricia Benner are examples of nurse scholars whose work reflects a view that the individual is different from and greater than the sum of the parts. Table 3-2 describes the concept of person as reflected in the work of several nurse theorists.

TABLE 3-2
Theoretic ideas about the person

Author	Concepts of person
Joyce Travelbee (1966)	A single human being, family, or community whose illness experience has unique meaning
Virginia Henderson (1966)	Mind and body are inseparable. No two individuals are alike; each is unique. The individual's basic needs are reflected in 14 components of basic nursing care.
Martha Rogers (1970)	Unitary human being is viewed as an energy field, the boundaries of which extend beyond the discernible mass of the human body. There are five unifying assumptions about the life process: (1) unified wholeness, (2) openness, (3) unidirectionality, (4) pattern and organization, and (5) sentience.
Dorothea Orem (1971)	The individual is an integrated whole composed of an internal physical, psychologic, and social nature with varying degrees of self-care ability.
Imogene King (1971)	Individuals are viewed as (1) reacting beings, (2) time-oriented beings, and (3) social beings, with the ability to perceive, think, feel, choose, set goals, and make decisions.
Patricia Benner and Judith Wrubel (1989)	The person is a self-interpreting being engaged in the world. Engagement is possible because of the human capacities of embodied intelligence, culturally acquired meanings, concern, and direct involvement in or grasp of a situation.

Emergence of nursing theory

Society and environment

The concept of society and environment is consistently viewed as central to the discipline of nursing. These concepts are not addressed as fully in some writings as in others. Several nursing theories deal with the concept of society and view society, or culture, as a critical interacting force shaping the individual (Table 3-3). The environment was central for Nightingale in her concepts of nursing. Nightingale believed that the primary focus for nursing was to alter the physical environment to place the human body in the best possible condition for the reparative processes of nature to occur. Several early contemporary nurse authors gave less emphasis to environment per se or viewed it as encompassing the notion of society, sometimes using the word "society" to include environment. However, the concept of environment has reemerged as a significant one, particularly in the work of Martha Rogers and theorists who build on her ideas.

Health

The concept of health is usually identified as the purpose or goal of nursing. Nightingale stated "the same laws of health or of nursing, for in reality they are the same, obtain among the well as among the sick" (Nightingale, 1969, p. 9). Contemporary nursing theories are remarkably congruous with this early conceptualization. Some theories and models are based on a conceptualization of a health-illness continuum, and nursing's purpose is to assist

TABLE 3-3

Theoretic ideas about society and environment

Author	Concepts of society/environment
Florence Nightingale (1860)	Environment is the central concept. It is viewed as all external conditions and influences affecting life and the development of the organism. The major emphasis is on warmth, effluvia (odors), noise, and light.
Joyce Travelbee (1966)	Environment is the context in which human-to-human relatedness is established.
Myra Levine (1967)	Society is viewed as the total environment of the individual, including family, significant others, and the nurse.
Sister Callista Roy (1976)	Environment constantly interacts with the individual and determines, in part, adaptation level. Stimuli originate in the environment.

TABLE 3-4
Theoretic ideas about health

Author	Terms related to health
Lydia Hall (1966)	Self actualization, self love
Virginia Henderson (1966)	Independent function
Myra Levine (1967)	Maintaining holism/conservation
Dorthea Orem (1971)	Self-care agency
Josephine Paterson and Loretta Zderad (1976)	Authentic awareness
Sister Callista Roy (1976)	Continual adaptation
Margaret Newman (1986)	Expanding consciousness

the ill client to achieve the highest degree of health possible. Other nurse authors view the concept of health as something more than, or different from, the absence of disease. It exists independently from illness or disease. In these views, health is a dynamic process that changes with time and varies according to life circumstances. Some authors view the health process as interdependent with circumstances of the environment, whereas others view the health process as something that originates with the individual (Smith, 1983).

In an attempt to deal more specifically with ideas related to health, several nurse authors avoid using the terms "health" and "illness." An example is use of the term "conserving holism." This concept directs nurses to focus on the totality of a person's situation rather than on the typical parameters that have come to be commonly known as "health." Table 3-4 identifies some of the terms that nurses have used in constructing their theoretic ideas about health. These terms suggest ideas that more specifically reflect nursing's concerns and de-emphasize the focus on disease or illness.

THE DISCIPLINE OF NURSING: PHILOSOPHY OF DEVELOPMENT OF NURSING KNOWLEDGE

A discipline is characterized by collective knowledge development among persons within a common interest area. One trait that distinguishes a discipline from other social groups is the purpose for developing theory and knowledge. Groups of people who have common interests such as bridge clubs or church congregations are social groups. People in these groups sometimes take on projects that involve improving their knowledge and skill related to specific interests, but their primary purpose for forming the group is not to develop new knowledge. An occupational group is formed by individuals who share certain job-related skills and knowledge. Hairdressers, office workers, or real estate agents constitute occupational groups. People in these groups engage in learning activities to acquire and update skills and understandings. Groups whose purpose is to produce new theory and knowledge within an area of inquiry are known as disciplines. Professions such as social work, nursing, or medicine are composed of people who practice and people who develop new knowledge to be used in the practice. Scholars who create knowledge also select and create knowledge development methods that are suited to the requirements of the practice and propose the standards by which the knowledge of the discipline is judged to be worthwhile (Donaldson and Crowley, 1978). Early nursing theorists and philosophers provided a significant foundation from which nursing has evolved as a discipline. Their writings formed the characteristics of nursing's knowledge. Within this common frame of reference, there is a great deal of room for diversity of views. This diversity makes possible the creation of new and more useful ideas as the times and contexts of the practice of nursing change.

The nature of key nursing concepts and holism

A major philosophic dilemma in the development of new knowledge is how to determine what kinds of knowledge and approaches to developing knowledge are most valuable. This dilemma is most evident when the nature of primary concepts within the discipline of nursing are considered. A key example is the concept that nursing has of the individual as a holistic being. The methods of science, as well as the criteria by which the methods are judged as being adequate, have traditionally been based on objective observation of discrete elements, deliberately isolated from the whole.

The concept of a holistic *person* means that nothing is reduced to discrete elements or isolated from its context (Francis, 1980; Newman, 1979; Winstead-Fry, 1980, Kramer, 1990). The concepts of *health* that have emerged in nursing imply a movement or development toward wholeness. The concept that the totality of the *environment* and the place of the person in *society* contributes to wholeness indicates that nursing must view the individual and the environment as an integral whole.

Moccia (1988) observed that choosing methods for developing nursing knowledge is not based solely on technical considerations. Rather, the choices we make in method represent significant philosophic issues that concern the nature of what it means to be human. From this perspective, nursing cannot "patch" traditional scientific methods together with newer methods of inquiry and thereby achieve methods that are consistent with a view of human wholeness. She states:

> The dilemma that has finally been uncovered by the methods debate is whether science and professionalism are designed and/or able to serve humanity or whether they will instead serve those with the power to define and control what is meant by science and professionalism. . . . If the goal of [nursing] practice is to assist people in developing potential that is uniquely theirs, then research is needed that will give researchers and providers information to enhance the depth and complexity of their understanding of individual instances. The choice is how to become more fully engaged in the lives of those who are to receive nursing care rather than more completely distanced from their daily activities (Moccia, 1988, p. 7).

Several nurse scholars have proposed methods or approaches to the development of nursing knowledge that are consistent with the philosophic meanings of the concept of holism. Criticisms of the methods and approaches of traditional science that appeared in nursing literature have clarified the essential problems, making way for proposals for alternative methods (Bramwell, 1984; Engel, 1984; Benner, 1985; Moccia, 1985; Jacobs, 1986; Stevens, 1989).

Margaret Newman (1979) proposed that a holistic approach requires identifying patterns that reflect the whole. Patricia Benner and Judith Wrubel (1989) proposed a phenomenologic/hermeneutic method of inquiry that rests on the meaning of experience as primary to all else, grounding the view of the person within that total context and the meanings of that context.

The methods that we propose to integrate the personal, esthetic, ethical, and empiric patterns of knowing reflect how we address the inclusion of methods that are congruous with holism. Integration of knowledge enables choices that are congruous with the tenets of holism.

THE CONTEXTS OF THEORY DEVELOPMENT

Nursing history creates specific circumstances and contexts that influence the development of theory. These include professional, individual, and societal values and resources. Table 3-5 lists values and resources that continue to influence the development of theory in nursing.

Values

Individual values include an individual's commitment, motives, personal philosophy, beliefs, and priorities. Professional values are beliefs and ideologies that are generally held in common by members of the profession and are used to guide professional action. Professional values are expressed in

TABLE 3-5
Values and resources that influence theory development

Whip lines	Examples of specific factors
VALUES	
Individual	Commitment to the discipline
	Philosophy of nursing
	Motives
	World view of philosophy
	Priorities for action
Professional	Commitment to development of knowledge
	Code of ethics
	Standards for practice
	Standards for human subjects in research
	Willingness to challenge social traditions
	Priorities for allocating the resources of the professional group
Societal	Cultural mores
	Ethical codes
	Priorities for allocating resources
RESOURCES	
Individual	Cognitive style
	Intellectual ability
	Personality
	Life-style and setting
	Educational background
	Life experience
	Economic power
Professional	Educational requirements for members
	Body of literature
	Methodologies and instrumentation
	Group profile in relation to education, economic power, political influence
Societal	Settings for practice, education, and research
	Funding for the discipline's activities
	Material requirements

formal statements issued by professional groups in the form of codes, standards of practice, and ethical theory. Professional values are also reflected in repeated themes that occur in the literature and in the collective actions taken by professional organizations.

Societal values are ideologies expressed through societal choices, sanctions, and mores during a given period in history. When individual, professional, and societal values are basically congruous, there is relative stability, and new insights tend to build on what is already established as knowledge in the discipline. When individual, professional, or societal values conflict with or challenge one another, the potential exists for creating fundamental change in knowledge and in practice.

Resources

Resources can also be viewed as individual, professional, and societal. Individual resources include the natural and acquired talents shared among members of the discipline, including cognitive style, intellectual abilities, life circumstances, and educational preparation. The collective membership of the discipline forms the professional resources that support ongoing theory development. Examples of professional resources include a growing body of literature, the educational attainments of members of the profession and the nature of that education, as well as methodologies and instrumentation available for theory development.

Societal resources are those circumstances, materials, space, and funds acquired by the profession from the society at large. Acquisition of societal resources depends on features of the society, as well as those of the profession. For example, political influence is required to obtain funds, materials, and space to carry out the activities of the discipline. If the political system of society reflects priorities other than those that concern nursing, societal resources are less available to nursing than to other groups that reflect those priorities.

The problem of allocating resources illustrates the circular relationship between resources and values. Politics involves value decisions about who does and does not deserve the resources of society. If, as the course of history shows, women scientists are consistently denied the resources of society, the ability of women to influence value decisions is lessened. Nursing is a group comprised mostly of women (a professional resource) within a societal context that devalues women as scientists. This fact influences the profession's ability to exert influence on society at large and gain access to resources. The contemporary women's movement is creating a stimulus for recognizing societal restrictions on nursing as a sex-segregated occupation and the effects of systematic oppression of nurses and nursing (Greenleaf, 1980; Roberts,

1983). Feminist theory, which shares many of the traits of nursing theory, provides a perspective for changing social values and shifting social resources. Feminism places on society an urgent demand for a values transformation that is consistent with nursing's vision of health, the health care system, and nursing (Chinn and Wheeler, 1985). As women's experience is increasingly valued as a resource for developing knowledge, the resulting values conflict between traditional views, and the new values will open avenues for change.

EVOLVING DIRECTIONS IN NURSING THEORY

In the early 1950s efforts to represent nursing theoretically produced broad conceptualizations of nursing practice. These broad conceptual models or frameworks (in our view, also theories) proliferated during the 1960s and 1970s and are growing and changing. These early theories represented an ideal for nursing—the "oughts" of nursing. They suggested the nature of the person, society and environment, and health. They described the nurses' role and the philosophic foundations of the profession. They challenged the reality of nursing practice through their idealistic stance about nursing.

Although the broad conceptual models and frameworks were not developed using research processes, they did provide real direction for nursing by focusing on a general ideal of practice that served as a guide for research and curricula. Table 3-6 presents a chronologic list of nurse theorists who have produced broad conceptualizations of nursing from the 1950s to the present. The order of listing is determined by the first major published work. Many of the women who appear early in the chronology continue to actively publish in the nursing literature. Some of the nurse theorists listed later had a much earlier influence within nursing by communicating their ideas in professional circles before they were published. The table also includes our view of the key emphasis of each theorist's work. An interpretive summary of the writings of each theorist in the table can be found the Appendix.

Over time the focus of these theories has changed significantly to parallel changes in society. Systems theory had widespread acceptance in the biologic and social sciences during the 1960s. The influence of systems theory can be particularly noted in the work of Imogene King, Dorothy Johnson, and Sister Callista Roy. The theories of Martha Rogers, Rosemarie Parse, and Margaret Newman reflect theoretic perspectives in modern physics that move beyond earlier system concepts of equilibrium. Other theorists who continue to write also have changed their perspectives over time. These changes may not be directly linked to changes in the social/political context within which nursing theories develop, but they may reflect evolution of the theorist's

TABLE 3-6

Chronology of conceptual models in nursing (1952-1981)

Year of first major publication	Theorist	Key emphasis
1952	Hildegard E. Peplau	Interpersonal process is maturing force for personality.
1960	Faye G. Abdellah Irene L. Beland Almeda Martin Rugh V. Matheney	Patient's problems determine nursing care.
1961	Ida Jean Orlando	Interpersonal process alleviates distress.
1964	Ernestine Weidenbach	Helping process meets needs through art of individualizing care.
1966	Lydia E. Hall	Nursing care is person directed toward self-love.
1966	Joyce Travelbee	Meaning in illness determines how people respond.
1967	Myra E. Levine	Holism is maintained by conserving integrity.
1970	Martha E. Rogers	Person-environment are energy fields that evolve negentropically.
1971	Dorothea E. Orem	Self-care maintains wholeness.
1971	Imogene M. King	Transactions provide a frame of reference toward goal setting.
1974	Sr. Callista Roy	Stimuli disrupt an adaptive system.
1976	Josephine G. Paterson Loretta T. Zderad	Nursing is an existential experience of nurturing.
1978	Madeleine M. Leininger	Caring is universal and varies transculturally.
1979	Jean Watson	Caring is moral ideal: mind-body-soul engagement with another.
1979	Margaret A. Newman	Disease is a clue to preexisting life patterns.
1980	Dorothy E. Johnson	Subsystems exist in dynamic stability.
1981	Rosemarie Rizzo Parse	Indivisible beings and environment cocreate health.

ideas. Theorists whose theoretic perspective changes with successive publications include Sister Callista Roy, Jean Watson, and Madeleine Leininger.

These broad theories can be grouped according to some unique trait or feature. For example, Sisca-Riehl (1989) categorizes theories into "developmental" and "interaction" types, implying that these concepts are related to nursing. Common themes can also be seen in the influence of one theorist's ideas on others. Ernestine Weidenbach and Ida Jean Orlando both focus on the importance of meeting patient needs. Although from a different perspective, Leininger and Watson emphasize the concept of caring as a central focus for nursing. When theories are grouped, regardless of the category, central concepts or images for nursing are formed.

How theory is being defined in nursing is changing. Changing definitions reflect shifts in defining what theory is and how it is created. This evolution makes it difficult to decide exactly what counts as a "theory." Doctoral programs in nursing are increasing. More and more, nurses are being educated to conduct research and create theory. As numbers of doctorally prepared nurses are employed in nursing, the potential for creating theory based on and evolving from research increases.

Today nursing theory at the midrange level is being developed and is a significant and valuable presence. Creating midrange theory relies on linking theory directly with research or generating theory from research. In either approach, research and theory interact to modify and shape both. Whereas broad conceptual frameworks provide general ideals for practice, midrange theory can be used to more directly guide care. Some examples of midrange concepts that currently form a focus for theory development in nursing are: social support, prenatal maternal attachment, chronic fatigue, stress-coping, and pain control. Theory is also developing around midrange concepts that do not directly pertain to clinical care such as the role of women as nurses, administrative practice, and professionalism; this increasing activity is changing the nature of theory-research and theory-practice links and redefining theory.

Major approaches to defining nursing are being developed and used but may not be identified as theory. Nursing diagnosis taxonomies are a prime example. The widespread recognition of nursing diagnoses represents the enactment of a theoretic position about nursing. The ANA policy statement is also a theory-like formulation that has had a significant influence on nursing. It formulates a value stance about nursing much like those found in the broad conceptual frameworks listed in Table 3-6.

Theoretic activity is also increasing in relation to the ethical basis of nursing practice. Although early conceptual models and frameworks followed the scientific-empiric̆ form of theory construction, they embodied normative goals that were grounded in an ethic of nursing. Within nursing there is increasing recognition of the need to develop conceptualizations of ethics as ways of being rather than as sets of selectively applied rules and guidelines for practice.

CONCLUSION

In this chapter we have presented an overview of the history from which theory in nursing evolves. The values and resources that influence theory development are rooted in history. The history of nursing determines the nature of nursing's knowledge, as well as how knowledge in nursing develops. The history, values, and resources of nursing have been influenced by cultural and societal circumstances that closely parallel the status and role of women. As early theorists in nursing developed a sense of community and scholarship, they expressed differences and commonalities that have influenced more recent theoretic developments. A perspective of history and an understanding of values and resources affecting the development of theory make it possible to refine understandings of what theory is. In Chapter 4 we will examine various definitions of theory that have been published in nursing literature and develop a definition that is consistent with nursing's key concepts and patterns of knowing.

REFERENCES

Abdellah FG: The nature of nursing science, Nurs Res 18(5):390–393, 1969.

Abdellah FG et al: Patient-centered approaches to nursing, New York, 1960, The Macmillan Co.

Ashley JA: Hospitals, paternalism, and the role of the nurse, New York, 1976, Teacher's College Press.

Barnard KE and Neal MV: Maternal-child nursing research: review of the past and strategies for the future, Nurs Res 26(1):193–200, 1977.

Benner P: From novice to expert: excellence and power in clinical nursing practice, Menlo Park, 1984, Addison-Wesley.

Benner P: Quality of life: a phenomenological perspective on explanation, prediction, and understanding in nursing science, Adv Nurs Sci 8(1):1–14, 1985.

Benner P and Wrubel J: The primacy of caring, Menlo Park, 1989, Addision-Wesley.

Bramwell L: Use of life history in pattern identification and health promotion, Adv Nurs Sci 7(12):37–44, 1984.

Chinn PL and Wheeler CE: Feminism and nursing, Nurs Outlook 33(2):74–77, 1985.

Christy TE: Portrait of a leader, Nurs Outlook 6(6):72–75, 1969.

Dennis KE and Prescott PA: Florence Nightingale: yesterday, today, and tomorrow, Adv Nurs Sci 7(2):66–81, 1985.

Dickoff J and James P: A theory of theories: a position paper, Nurs Res 17(3):197–203, 1968.

Dickoff J and James P: Clarity to what end? Nurs Res 20(6):499–502, 1971.

Dickoff J, James P, and Wiedenbach E: Theory in a practice discipline. I. Practice-oriented theory, Nurs Res 17(5):415–435, 1968.

Donaldson SK and Crowley DM: The discipline of nursing, Nurs Outlook 26(2):113–120, 1978.

Ellis R: Commentary on "Toward a clearer understanding of the concept of nursing theory," Nurs Res 20(6):493–494, 1971.

Engel NS: On the vicissitudes of health appraisal, Adv Nurs Sci 7(1):12–23,1984.

Fawcett J: The relationship between theory and research: a double helix, Adv Nurs Sci 1(1):49–62, 1978.

Flaskerud JH and Halloran EJ: Areas of agreement in nursing theory development, Adv Nurs Sci 3(1):1–7, 1980.

Folta JR: Obfuscation or clarification: a reaction to Walker's concept of nursing theory, Nurs Res 20(6):496–499, 1971.

Francis G: Gesellshaft and the hospital: is total care a misnomer? Adv Nurs Sci 2(4):9–13, 1980.

Greenleaf, NP: Sex-segregated occupations: relevance for nursing, Adv Nurs Sci 2(3):23–38, 1980.

Hall LE: A center for nursing, Nurs Outlook 11(11):805–806, 1963.

Hall LE: Nursing: what is it? Can Nurse 60(2):150–154, 1964.

Hall LE: Another view of nursing care and quality. In Straub KM and Parker KS, editors: Continuity in patient care: the role of nursing, Washington, DC, 1966, Catholic University Press, pp 47–60.

Hardy ME: Perspectives on nursing theory, Adv Nurs Sci 1(1):37–48, 1978.

Henderson V: The nature of nursing, Am J Nurs 64(8):62–68, 1964.

Henderson V: The nature of nursing, New York, 1966, The Macmillan Co.

Hughes L: The public image of the nurse, Adv Nurs Sci 2(3):55–72, 1980.

Jacobs, MK: Can nursing theory be tested? In Chinn PL, editor: Methodological issues in nursing, Rockville, 1986, Aspen Publications, Inc.

Johnson DE: The behavioral system model for nursing. In Riehl JP and Roy SR C, editors: Conceptual models for nursing practice ed 2, New York, 1980, Appleton-Century-Crofts, pp 207–216.

Kalisch PA and Kalisch BJ: The advance of American nursing, Boston, 1978, Little, Brown, & Co.

Kelly LY: Dimensions of professional nursing, ed 5, New York, 1985, The Macmillan Co.

King IM: Toward a theory for nursing: general concepts of human behavior, New York, 1971, John Wiley & Sons.

Kramer MK: Holistic nursing: implications for knowledge development and utilization. In Chaska NL: The nursing profession: turning points, St. Louis, 1990, Mosby-Year Book, Inc, pp 245–254.

Krueter FR: What is good nursing care? Nurs Outlook 5(5):302–304, 1957.

Leininger MM: Doctoral programs for nurses: trends, questions, and projected plans, Nurs Res 25(3):201–210, 1976.

Levine ME: The four conservation principles of nursing, Nurs Forum, 6(1):93–98, 1967.

Lovell MC: The politics of medical deceptions: challenging the trajectory of history, Adv Nurs Sci 2:73–86, 1980.

Melosh B: The physician's hand: work culture and conflict in American nursing, Philadelphia, 1982, Temple University Press.

Moccia, P: A further investigation of "dialectical thinking as a means of understanding systems-in-development: relevance to Roger's principles," Adv Nurs Sci 7(4):33–38, 1985.

Moccia PA: A critique of compromise: beyond the methods debate, Adv Nurs Sci 10(4):1–9, 1988.

Newman MA: Theory development in nursing, Philadelphia, 1979, FA Davis Co.

Nightingale F: Notes on nursing: what it is and what is is not, New York, 1969, Dover Publications (originally published in 1860 by D. Appleton and Co).

Nightingale F: Cassandra, Old Westbury, NY, 1980, The Feminist Press, (introduction by M. Stark & Epilogue by C. MacDonald).

Orem DE: Nursing: concepts of practice, New York, 1971, McGraw-Hill Book Co, Inc.

Orlando IJ: The dynamic nurse-patient relationship: function, process, and principles, New York, 1961, GP Putnam's Sons.

Parse RR: Man-living-health: a theory of nursing, New York, 1981, John Wiley & Sons.

Theory and nursing: A systematic approach

Paterson JG and Zderad LT: Humanistic nursing, New York, 1976, John Wiley & Sons; published by National League for Nursing, 1988.

Reverby SM: Ordered to care: The dilemma of American nursing, 1850–1945, New York, 1987, Cambridge University Press.

Roberts S: Oppressed group behavior: implications for nursing, Adv Nurs Sci 5(4):21–30, 1983.

Rogers ME: An introduction to the theoretical basis of nursing, Philadelphia, 1970, FA Davis Co.

Roy, SR C: Introduction to nursing: an adaptation model, Englewood Cliffs, 1976, Prentice-Hall, Inc.

Sanger M: Margaret Sanger, an autobiography, New York, 1971, Dover Publications (originally published in 1938 by WW Norton).

Silverstein NG: Lillian Wald at Henry Street, 1893–1895, Adv Nurs Sci 7(2):1–12, 1985.

Sisca-Riehl JP, editor: Conceptual models for nursing practice, ed 3, New York, 1989, Appleton-Lange.

Smith JA: The idea of health: implications for the nursing professional, New York, 1983, Teachers College Press.

Stevens PE: A critical social reconceptualization of environment in nursing: implications for methodology, Adv Nurs Sci 11(4):56–68, 1989.

Tooley SA: The life of Florence Nightingale, New York, 1905, The Macmillan Co.

Travelbee J: Interpersonal aspects of nursing, Philadelphia, 1966, FA Davis Co.

Travelbee J: Interpersonal aspects of nursing, ed 2, Philadelphia, 1971, FA Davis Co.

Wald LD: The house of Henry Street, New York, 1971, Dover Publications, (originally published in 1915 by Holt, Rinehart, and Winston, Inc).

Walker, LO: Toward a clearer understanding of the concept of nursing theory, Nurs Res 20(5):428–435, 1971.

Walker LO: Rejoinder to commentary: toward a clearer understanding of the concept of nursing theory, Nurs Res 21(1):59–62, 1972.

Watson J: Nursing: the philosophy and science of caring, Boston, 1979, Little, Brown, & Co.

Watson J: Nursing: human science and human care, Norwalk, Conn, 1985, Appleton-Century-Crofts.

Whall AL: Congruence between existing theories of family functioning and nursing theories, Adv Nurs Sci 3(1):59–67, 1980.

Wheeler CE: The American Journal of Nursing and the socialization of a profession, 1900–1920, Adv Nurs Sci 7(2):20–34, 1985.

Wiedenbach E: Clinical nursing: a helping art, New York, 1964, Springer Publishing Co, Inc.

Winstead-Fry P: The scientific method and its impact on holistic health, Adv Nurs Sci 2(4):1–7, 1980.

Woodham-Smith C: Florence Nightingale: 1820–1910, New York, 1983, Atheneum.

Wooldridge PJ: Meta-theories of nursing: a commentary on Dr. Walker's article, Nurs Res 20(6):494–495, 1971.

Yura H and Torres G: Today's conceptual frameworks within baccalaureate nursing programs, Faculty Curriculum Development, Part III, New York, 1975, National League for Nursing.

4

Nursing theory: an examination of the concept

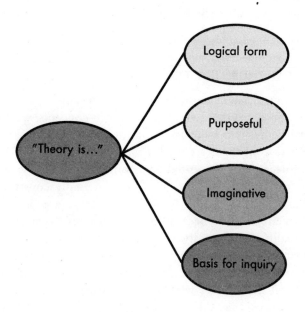

The word "theory" has many meanings. From our perspective, nursing theory need not be limited to any one theoretic trait. A definition that is useful for characterizing nursing theory must be broad enough to include diverse types of theory.

What exactly is nursing theory? There are several ways to answer this seemingly simple question. In Chapters 1 and 2 we reviewed the dimensions and forms of empirically patterned knowledge and discussed a broad definition of theory, which provided a general understanding of the nature of theory and its contribution to the whole of knowing. In this chapter, we examine four distinct definitions of theory and a range of traits that characterize theory. From this, we propose a definition of theory useful for nursing. Our definition reflects the range of theory development processes and outcomes that we believe are necessary for the growth of nursing knowledge.

COMPLEXITY OF ABSTRACT CONCEPTS

The word "theory" has multiple meanings because it represents a very abstract concept. Since theory is also built from concepts, we begin this discussion of what theory is by considering the nature of concepts.

We define a concept as a complex mental formulation of empiric experience. All concepts can be located on a continuum from the empiric (more directly experienced) to the abstract (more mentally constructed) (Jacox, 1974; Kaplan, 1964). In one sense, all concepts are both empiric and abstract. They are empiric because they are formed from encounters with perceptible reality. They are abstract because they are cognitive representations of what is perceptually experienced. Concepts differ in the ways in which they directly relate to perceptible reality. Some concepts are formed from very direct experiences with reality, whereas others are formed from indirect experiences. Fig. 4-1 illustrates this continuum. Relatively empiric concepts are ideas that are formed from direct observations of objects, properties, or events. As concepts become more abstract, they can only be experienced indirectly. The most abstract concepts encompass a complex network of subconcepts that can only be inferred. Concepts formed about objects such as a "cup" or properties such as "hot" are examples of highly empiric concepts because the object or property that represents the idea (empiric indicator) can be directly experienced through the senses. A relatively empiric property such as gender can also be observed directly by noting the primary and secondary sexual characteristics that identify a person as male or female. Properties such as height and weight can be measured using

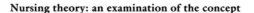

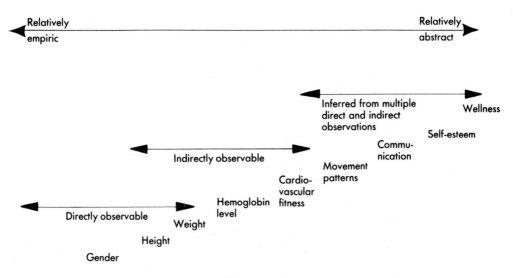

FIG. 4-1
Example of empiric-abstract continuum.

standardized instruments. Since the measurement is relatively direct, height and weight are relatively empiric concepts.

As concepts become more abstract, their reality basis and their empiric indicators become less concrete and less directly measurable. Assessment of an abstract concept depends increasingly on indirect means. Although an indirect assessment or observation is different in kind from direct measurement, it is considered to be a reasonable indicator of the concept. "Hemoglobin level" is representative of a concept that cannot be directly observed but can be indirectly "seen" with the aid of laboratory instruments. This type of measurement depends on more complex and less direct forms of instrumentation.

Cardiovascular fitness is an example of a concept that is mid-range on the empiric-abstract continuum. Concepts increase in complexity in this range, and several empiric indicators must be assessed. Because no object such as "cardiovascular fitness" exists, definition is required if we are to know what it is. Even though definitions for less empirically based concepts are thoughtfully formulated, they are arbitrary, because many different definitions could be chosen. As concepts become increasingly abstract, definitions become more dependent on the theoretic meaning of the concept and the purpose for defining it.

"Self esteem" is an example of a highly abstract concept for which there are no direct measures. The instruments or tools that are developed to indirectly assess "self-esteem" depend on theoretic definitions serving a specific purpose. An instrument or tool developed to assess or measure an abstract concept such as "self esteem" is built on multiple behavioral responses that are thought to be associated with that concept. Ideas about these responses are set forth in a theory or may generate from concept clarification (see Chapter 5). Each behavioral trait contained in the tool can be designated as an empiric indicator. When the composite behaviors are built into an assessment tool, it is usually a more adequate indicator for the abstract concept than any one behavior taken alone. The composite score obtained from the tool is then considered to be a measurement constructed as an empiric indicator.

Highly abstract concepts are sometimes called constructs. Constructs are the most complex type of concept on the empiric-abstract continuum. These concepts include ideas with a reality base so abstract that it is "constructed" from multiple sources of direct and indirect evidence. An example of a construct is "wellness." Wellness exists almost solely as an idea. Fig. 4-1 illustrates the idea that highly abstract concepts are constructed from other concepts. All of the concepts shown on the continuum (as well as others) can be included in the concept of "wellness."

Some abstract concepts have little meaning outside the context of a theory. Often ideas that are unique to the theoretic context cannot be meaningfully used outside the theory. For example, Levine (1967) coined the word "trophicogenic" to mean "nurse-induced illness." Rogers (1970) discussed three "principles of homeodynamics. Rogers' term "homeodynamics" is a combination of the Latin root word "homeo" meaning "similar to" or "like" and the common English term "dynamics" meaning "pattern of change or growth." The reader can infer the meaning "change processes" for the term "homeodynamics," which is consistent with Rogers' intent.

Abstract concepts may also acquire additional meaning through gradual transfer into common language usage. Freud's concept of "ego" is an example. Once the word "ego" had no common meaning outside of Freud's theory, but today, with gradual changes in its meaning and broad usage outside the theory, everyone knows the meaning of "a big ego."

Although it is usually not necessary to identify where concepts fit on an empiric-abstract continuum, it is important to understand that concepts vary in the degree to which they are connected to empiric reality and to which their meaning is mentally constructed.

Defining and understanding concepts

When you begin to study something abstract like "theory," it is natural to wonder why it is difficult to grasp the meaning of the term and understand the concept. It is helpful to recognize that even highly empiric concepts like "cup" are not easily understood and defined. To illustrate, conjure up an image of a cup. What you have done is to create an image of the object in your mind—you have brought into awareness a concept. Now describe the image you have in your mind's eye. Your definition might be something like this:

> **cup** A hard-surfaced, hollow cylinder, closed on one end, with a small handle attached to the cylindric surface, that is often used for drinking.

Note that the cup defined above is for drinking, but other "cup" images are possible. A cup can mean other things as illustrated in the phrases "to cup a hand," "to offer a cup of cheer," and "the golf ball dropped into the cup." When different meanings for cup are suggested, where you would place the concept on the empiric-abstract continuum changes. Placing a concept on the continuum requires that you know its definition or how it is being used. A "cup of cheer," unlike the drinking cup, cannot be directly experienced but can be inferred from behaviors in a cultural context. The use of the word "cup" as in "a cup of cheer" represents a more abstract concept than use of the word in reference to an ordinary drinking cup.

In the development of language, once a word representing an object has been established, the object may change, and ambiguity develops about the use of the term. For example, the term "cup" can be used to refer to a stoneware mug or a china teacup. Each object is quite different, and they are found in different social contexts, but the definition given above for each is adequate. To be more specific, the definition would need to include additional features of the cup that are appropriate to the context in which it is used, material that the cup is made of, or other objects that accompany the use of the cup.

To further illustrate the difficulty of defining even concrete concepts, omit from the original definition of "cup" the feature of a handle. The definition now reads:

> **cup** A hard-surfaced, hollow cylinder closed on one end, often used for drinking.

You can now appreciate the significance of the handle for distinguishing this object from a glass. When this portion of the definition is omitted, the dimensions and composition of the object, as well as the context of usage, become important for determining whether the object is a cup or a glass. A cup may be defined as being shorter and wider than a glass, and differentiation between them would rely on their physical dimensions.

Sometimes distinctions between objects are not important, and a definition that includes a wide range of meaning is adequate. Imagine an opaque, styrofoam drinking vessel that holds about 8 ounces, has no handle, is shaped like a section of a cone, and is closed on the narrow end. Is this object a "cup" or a "glass?" For some people it is a cup, for others a glass, and for still others it matters little, and it is both! Without detailed definitions for both the concepts of cup and glass, there is no basis for distinguishing between the two, and, even with definitions, the decision about which label to use is arbitrary and depends on the purpose.

Ambiguities in definitions

Ambiguities exist in all definitions, even for those of very concrete realities. For example, our definition of the word "cup" does not specify how or where the handle is placed on the cylindric surface. These ambiguities are greatly magnified when defining highly abstract concepts. Defining abstract realities requires a tolerance of ambiguity. Choices must be made about which empiric reality is represented in an abstract concept and which is not.

Because of its highly abstract nature, the word "theory" is defined in many different ways. The question often arises, "Is this a theory or a conceptual framework?" This question is reasonable, for one nurse's theory may be another's conceptual framework. Reasonable definitions are neither right nor wrong, and it may be difficult to decide about the best definition for a given purpose. Our aim is to present various definitions of this highly abstract concept, examine them for commonalties and differences, and present a definition for the term "theory" that is suited to our ideas about how theory develops in nursing.

COMPARATIVE ANALYSIS OF DEFINITIONS OF THEORY

In Chapter 2 we defined theory broadly as a "systematic abstraction of reality that serves some purpose." Theoretic purposes included the description, explanation, and prediction of empiric reality. Although this definition is not incorrect, it is broad and therefore not always helpful in understanding what theory is and how it is created. The phrase "systematic abstraction" suggests a product or outcome, as well as a series of thoughts, actions, or processes by which the outcomes are created. The definitions we examine here suggest the specific processes that are used to create the systematic abstraction processes. The definitions also suggest different possible outcomes when theory development processes are carried out.

Rose McKay: The form of theory development

Theory has been defined by McKay as a "logically interconnected set of confirmed hypotheses" (McKay, 1969, p. 394). This definition implies that reasoned thought, armchair style, that does not use confirmed hypotheses as raw material will not produce theory. The definition also implies that research processes are integral to the building of theory because confirmed hypotheses do not arise otherwise.

A hypothesis is a type of propositional statement. It is a single statement of a proposed relationship between two or more variables. Hypotheses can take several forms and still provide a basis for developing theory. A neutral hypothesis asserts that one variable (X) is related to a second variable (Y) or that one variable (X) changes in relation to another (Y) without indicating the direction of change. A directional hypothesis indicates the direction of association between variables where, as one variable (X) increases or decreases, a second (Y) also increases or decreases.

A confirmed hypothesis is a relationship statement for which there is research support. It can be either directional or neutral. Hypothesis testing requires that certain controls and procedures be adhered to and that statistical models be applied in the confirmation process. Thus a specific type of research is basic to the development of theory according to this definition of theory.

Most theory in nursing does not meet the requirements of the McKay definition, yet the definition is not wrong. In fact, it reflects a traditional notion of what theory is, particularly within the natural sciences (physics, chemistry, biology) and the formal sciences (logic and mathematics). In sciences in which phenomena obey natural laws or can be isolated from their context and controlled, it is possible to confirm hypotheses and logically interconnect them. In such sciences the range of variables is often narrow, and experimental research approaches are used so variables can be singularly added in a controlled environment and their effects on outcomes monitored. Control over the environment and the variables under study helps ensure that a hypothesis will be reliably confirmed or rejected.

In addition to requiring confirmed hypotheses for theory construction, the McKay definition implies that the hypotheses are connected using rules of logic. The logic may be either deductive or inductive. The following sections provide an overview of each of these forms of logic.

Deductive forms of logic. Deductive logic is a system of reasoning in which propositions—assertions of relationship—are interrelated in a consistent way. In deductive logic the logician begins with two premises as propositions (sometimes called axioms) and draws a conclusion, or a proposition, that is directly dependent on the premises. In logic the format used is fixed. "Format" refers to the structure of interrelationships among the premises and the conclusion without regard to the meaningfulness of the premises. It is possible to have a valid, or formally correct, logical argument that is not meaningful when compared with empiric experience.

Theory developed from application of deductive systems of logic is only as sound as the premises on which the argument is based. One form of deductive logic is:

> (premise) A is B.
> (premise) C is A.
> (conclusion) C is B.

The problem of reaching a sound conclusion occurs when concepts, representing human characteristics, are substituted for the letters. The problem of soundness of deductive logic can be illustrated with the following:

> (premise) Humans (A) use cups with handles (B).
> (premise) Infants (C) are humans (A).
> (conclusion) Infants (C) use cups with handles (B).

With substitutions of words representing selected concepts, the soundness of the conclusion is questionable, even though the form is valid. In this example the conclusion that infants use cups with handles cannot be justified as being consistent with empiric experience.

Confirmed hypotheses as premises are grounded in empiric reality. Because they are tested by research standards with imposed limitations, they can be considered valid. Confirmed hypotheses hold more potential for sound conclusions than unconfirmed hypotheses or suppositions. An example of a deductive argument in valid form and with reasonable premises (though unconfirmed) is as follows:

> (premise) Pregnant mammals retain fluid.
> (premise) Pregnant women are pregnant mammals.
> (conclusion) Pregnant women retain fluid.

The form of the argument is valid, and the first premise could be confirmed by research. Assuming confirmation of the first premise and the analytic (true by definition) nature of the second, the conclusion is likely to be more sound than one generated from untested premises.

Deductive logic is a way of reasoning. Its rules require a valid form of interrelationships between statements. Two or more relational statements are used to draw a concluding relational statement or proposition. Proposition, as a general term meaning an assertion of relationship between variables, can also be called a theorem. Premises, the statements on which the conclusion is based, may also be called hypotheses, suppositions, axioms, or simply propositions.

Laws may also arise from the application of deductive logic, especially in the science of mathematics. A law represents a highly generalizable assertion of relationship between variables. Laws can also be derived using other forms of logical thought.

Terms other than "axiom" and "theorem" for premises and conclusions in the empiric sciences (sciences other than logic and mathematics) reflect the tentative nature of propositions. In the empiric sciences premises and conclusions may be called hypotheses or suppositions.

Deductive conclusions can be used as premises in progressive logical arguments. This process links one logical idea to another, forming a type of theory. McKay's definition of theory limits theory to relationships that are confirmed research hypotheses. Some theory, however, develops by linking logical statements, which is known as "deducing hypotheses," implying that the theoretic relationships have not necessarily been confirmed empirically.

Although deductive systems of logic are valuable, there are certain hazards. Deduction based on suppositions or unconfirmed hypotheses may result in a valid but unsound argument. When the soundness of a conclusion is unknown, it may be erroneously assumed to be sound without serious challenge, especially if it seems reasonable. Deductive arguments based on confirmed hypotheses have a greater likelihood of achieving soundness, at least within the limits of their research testing. Although the empiric soundness of any conclusion may never be finally known, the utility of logical deductive conclusions for nursing increases if the premises have a degree of confirmation.

Inductive forms of logic. In the traditional view of science, deductive logic is the predominant form used in producing theory. However, the "logical" interconnections could also arise from the application of a second common system of logic: the inductive mode. This approach to theory development is being used in nursing in such approaches as grounded theory (Glaser and Strauss, 1967). In inductive logic the reasoning method relies on observing multiple particular instances and then combining those particulars into a larger whole. This can occur when the particular instances observed share common features and are part of a larger set of phenomena. The following example illustrates this approach: Assume that X1, X2, ... X5 are unique instances of a larger set Y, and that Y is associated with an effect or characteristic Z. The reasoning used is as follows:

> X1 is a member of set Y and is associated with Z.
> X2 is a member of set Y and is associated with Z.
> X3 is a member of set Y and is associated with Z.
> X4 is a member of set Y and is associated with Z.
> X5 is a member of set Y and is associated with Z.

Therefore X6, X7 ... Xn, or all X's are members of set Y and are associated with Z.

To substitute an empiric experience for the letter symbols in this illustration, let X be specific surgical techniques, let Y be surgical intervention, and let Z be postoperative pain. With these substitutions, the argument would proceed in the following manner:

> A dilatation and curettage as a surgical intervention is associated with postoperative pain.
> A laparotomy as a surgical intervention is associated with postoperative pain.
> A laser ablation as a surgical intervention is associated with postoperative pain.
> A burr hole as a surgical intervention is associated with postoperative pain.
> A closed reduction as a surgical intervention is associated with postoperative pain.
> Therefore all surgical interventions are associated with postoperative pain.

In this example the reasoning is that many specific instances of surgical techniques as surgical interventions are associated with the concept of postoperative pain. These surgical techniques share the empiric feature of being surgical interventions, which in turn are associated with postoperative pain.

Inductive reasoning would be considered sound when all specific instances of surgical techniques as surgical intervention (in our example X's) were observed to be associated with postoperative pain. A conclusion is drawn from the observation of specific instances of X's as subsets of surgical intervention associated with pain; and, when observations have been exhausted, the sets X and Y merge, and the argument is sound.

A second example serves to illustrate some pitfalls of inductive reasoning. In this example birds such as crows and ravens (X's) are specific instances of a larger set blackbirds (Y), and Z is the characteristic "ability to fly." The example is:

Nursing theory: an examination of the concept

A crow is a blackbird and can fly.
A raven is a blackbird and can fly.
A starling is a black bird and can fly.
A grackle is a black bird and can fly.
A vulture is a black bird and can fly.
Therefore all blackbirds can fly.

Since it is not possible to observe all instances of blackbirds that can fly, there is the possibility that the instance of a blackbird that cannot fly will be missed. If you have only seen crows, ravens, and starlings as blackbirds, you could easily conclude that all blackbirds can fly. If you chance to observe a black ostrich, your conclusion must be revised to accommodate the instance of a blackbird that cannot fly.

Inductive logic is limited because it is not possible to observe all instances of a specific event. This limitation must be considered when using inductive logic to generate theory.

In the example of surgical techniques as surgical interventions associated with pain, assume that the five instances cited were confirmed to be associated with postoperative pain. In inductive logic useful theory can be developed from observing and confirming that additional specific instances of surgical intervention were also associated with pain and concluding that "all" surgical interventions result in postoperative pain. It is not practical to show that all instances of surgical techniques as surgical intervention are associated with pain. The association can be shown to a degree of probability sufficient to develop useful theory, particularly when the context is limited.

Comparison of induction and deduction. Deductive logic is commonly referred to as reasoning from the general to the particular. Inductive logic is said to be reasoning from the particular to the general. In inductive logic particular instances are observed to be consistently part of a larger whole or set, and the set of particular instances is merged with that larger whole. This larger set can then be considered in relation to still another set of events or phenomena in another logical system.

In deductive logic the premises as starting points embody two variables that can be categorized in relation to each other as broad or specific. In the one example, pregnant mammals (a broad concept) were said to retain fluid (a specific concept). In the other premise, pregnant women were said to be pregnant mammals; that is, pregnant women specific were members of a broader class (pregnant mammals). The conclusion contains both of the specific variables: pregnant women retain fluid. In deductive logic the movement is from premises embodying broad and specific variables to a conclusion in which the variables are more specific.

Like most other words, deduction and induction have common meanings related to, but different from, their meaning within systems of logic. People often state that they deduce hypotheses from theory or deductively develop theory. These "deductions" are not the result of applying rules of logic but arise out of careful thought without specifically using a system of logic. Used like this, deduction implies that a more general theory was a source of specific hypotheses or relational statements.

With induction, people induce hypotheses and relationships by observing or experiencing an empiric reality and reaching some conclusion. These related meanings of induction and deduction should be noted because sometimes the terms refer to systems of logic and to rules and conventions for the ordering of reasoning. At other times the terms refer to a general approach to thinking, short of logical rules but similar in form.

McKay's definition of theory is useful because it focuses on the significance of logical thought and empiric confirmation in developing some forms of theory. However, as McKay notes, other definitions of theory that require less stringency in their approach are needed in nursing. Flexible approaches to theory development are valuable because nursing empirics must be consistent with the assumptions of human science. Nursing deals with a wide range of events that are complex and interconnected with countless other events. A strict and singular use of rules of logic and traditional scientific empiric confirmation is not consistent with nursing's concern with holistic beings whose actions are not governed by natural laws.

James Dickoff and Patricia James: The outcome of theory

Dickoff and James propose a definition of theory quite different from that of McKay. They define theory as "a conceptual system or framework invented to some purpose" (Dickoff and James, 1968, p. 198). Nursing is a service profession that has as one of its goals the promotion of health. Dickoff and James state that nursing must generate theory that will serve to achieve its goals or purposes. In this definition "purpose" is a key word, since theory is purpose oriented. In McKay's definition, even though clinical purpose is not explicitly addressed, some purpose—for example, explanation or prediction—would be identifiable for theory that is derived from research-tested hypotheses. Dickoff and James' definition requires the explicit articulation of a clear purpose or goal that directs the entire theory building effort (Dickoff and James, 1968; Dickoff, James, and Wiedenbach, 1968).

Invention is a second key idea within the Dickoff and James definition of theory. Invention implies that nursing creates the abstraction of reality that will achieve its purpose. The abstraction that is theory must be fashioned or made to happen, and its creation cannot occur apart from purpose. An analogy of a motor trip from the west coast to the eastern seaboard will illustrate this point. If you are in California and only know you want to move by car, you can get into the car and drive, and you will go somewhere. When you do this—get into a car and drive—you are only able to retrospectively describe a route taken. If you decide on a destination before beginning, you can invent and create the route as you proceed. One choice would be to wander around on the side roads and gather a lot of detailed experiences. Another choice would be to travel quickly on the freeway, gathering only those experiences that can be gleaned from the narrow vista perceived. According to Dickoff and James, theory building is a process of creating and inventing the pathway from among alternate choices that is guided by the destination. If there is no destination, it is only possible to give a retrospective account of features of the route. The Dickoff and James definition requires that a goal be stated and the way toward it created. Theory is deliberately created to achieve a purpose, and that purpose is value laden.

When theory is invented with some purpose in mind, theory development will occur in a way that is related to that purpose. Using this definition, the general form taken is a conceptual framework, and the processes of abstraction are varied. "Conceptual" means of or pertaining to concepts, whereas framework implies features of a structure or network. A conceptual framework is a network or structure of empirically based abstractions (concepts) that are represented by word symbols.

For Dickoff and James, theory develops on four levels: factor-isolating, factor-relating or situation-depicting, situation-relating, and situation-producing (Dickoff and James, 1968; Dickoff, James, and Wiedenbach, 1968). Level 1, factor-isolating, involves the naming or classification of phenomena. Level 2, factor-relating, requires correlating or associating factors in such a way that they become part of larger units that meaningfully depict a situation. Level 3, situation-relating, explains and predicts how situations are related. Level 4, situation-producing, requires sufficient knowledge about how and why situations are related so that, using theory as a guide, differing but valued situations can be produced (Dickoff and James, 1968, p. 200). Theory at each of the four levels is considered "theory."

For Dickoff and James the three ingredients of situation-producing theory (level 4) are: (1) goal content, (2) prescriptions, and (3) survey list (Dickoff, James, and Wiedenbach, 1968). The goal content conveys the purpose, whereas prescriptions and survey list comprise the major part of the conceptual framework. The invention involves devising and interrelating the conceptual framework components of prescriptions and survey list to achieve the purpose.

McKay's definition also implies the notion of level change as theory builds. If induction is the logical process used to build theory, theoretic levels change as concepts merge and become more inclusive. Deduction processes affect the level of theory by generating more particular knowledge as the logic proceeds. In contrast, for Dickoff and James the level of development does not necessarily relate to breadth of concepts, but classification of the level occurs according to how theoretic content builds to achieve the stated goal. According to Dickoff and James, research can be included in the theory development process. Although Dickoff and James imply that theory development progresses through four levels, all nursing efforts need not start at level 1. Whether implicit or explicit, theory at the situation-producing level builds on theory developed at lower levels.

In their definition, Dickoff and James use the phrase "conceptual framework." This includes as "theory" a wide variety of systematic abstractions developed by a variety of means and with varying precision. The survey list is an organized, empirically grounded guide to achieving a purpose. It assumes that prescriptions can never be complete. Survey lists embellish the prescriptions and aid goal achievement. The survey list is developed systematically using methods that are different from confirming hypotheses. Dickoff and James' requirement that an explicit clinical purpose be achieved differs from other definitions of theory. To Dickoff and James, situation-producing theory is essential in nursing; a clinical purpose must be clearly stated. Once the goal is determined and communicated, nurses then invent or create the path to the goal. Specific goal content increases the likelihood that descriptions, explanations, and predictions will be useful in nursing practice. Naming the goal content promotes theory development, which is clearly within nursing's area of concern and demystifies the theory development enterprise.

Jean Watson: The tentative nature of theory

Watson defines theory as: "An imaginative grouping of knowledge, ideas, and experience that are represented symbolically and seek to illuminate a given phenomena." (Watson, 1985, p. 1). Watson's purpose for theory is "seeking to illuminate a given phenomena." This implies a broad set of purposes for theory that could include understanding, as well as description, explanation, and prediction of nursing phenomena. This implies that the nurse can use theory to project and work toward goals. Dickoff and James, by contrast, require the articulation of a specific goal and the organization of the conceptualization so that goal achievement is approached. McKay's definition implies a general theoretic purpose. Because theory illuminates a given phenomena, Watson suggests that theory is bounded and limited.

The phrases "seeks to illuminate" and "imaginative grouping" are important in this definition because they make explicit the nature of theory as a tentative creation. The fact that theory is tentative is often implied in major writings on the subject, but is seldom directly acknowledged. The tentativeness of theory may not be obvious, for myths about theory perpetuate the notion that theory is somewhat final; since theory represents empiric reality—it is assumed to be reality. Science is based on a traditional view that truths exist independently from their discoverers. Discovered truths are assumed to proceed toward some ultimate and unchanging "final" truth. Consistent with emerging views, theory, research, and science are no longer thought to hold claim on eternal truths. Although theory may be a valuable representation of empiric experience, it is not final; it is tentative. The phrases "seeks to illuminate" and "imaginative grouping" in Watson's definition make explicit how "reality" is shaped by the imagination of the creator.

In Watson's definition the phrase "represented symbolically" is important because theory is an intermediate form of knowledge. Intermediate knowledge is conveyed through the use of symbols or words. For Watson, "knowledge, ideas, and experiences" are represented symbolically as theory, which integrates the personal values, perspective, and biases of its creator. This theory gives credence to personal ideas and experiences of nurses as a valuable source of knowledge.

Rosemary Ellis: Theory as a guide for inquiry

Ellis' definition of theory is: "conceptual and pragmatic principles forming a general frame of reference for a field of inquiry" (Ellis, 1968, p. 217). This definition of theory provides a reference point for guiding research inquiry and practice with assumed links between the two. Although not explicit in the definition, for Ellis a purpose of theory could be to achieve clinical goals, since theory provides a reference point for guiding inquiry. According to Ellis, if nursing practice provides the focus of inquiry, theory could help achieve a clinical purpose in the manner proposed by Dickoff and James. The wording of Ellis' definition suggests that research and theory are closely interrelated.

According to this definition, principles comprising theory form a conceptual framework that may or may not have strict logical interconnections. Theory as a means to guide inquiry implies that concepts are defined or used with a particular meaning, that certain assumptions are articulated, and that goals exist. This definition complements the other definitions with the idea that theory can function to guide research and inquiry.

A COMPREHENSIVE DEFINITION OF THEORY FOR NURSING

Although the preceding definitions are different, they share common features. Collectively they define a wide range of functions for theory. All are legitimate and accepted; each one focuses on a possible dimension of meaning. The four definitions are:

1. A logically interconnected set of confirmed hypotheses (McKay)
2. A conceptual system or framework invented to some purpose (Dickoff and James)
3. An imaginative grouping of knowledge, ideas, and experience that are represented symbolically and seek to illuminate a given phenomena (Watson)
4. A coherent set of hypothetic, conceptual, and pragmatic principles that form a general frame of reference for a field of inquiry (Ellis)

Beliefs about the nature of theory arise in part from the various fields of inquiry from which nursing knowledge is developed. Some nursing theorists come from educational traditions in which the ideal theory was that logically linked to sets of confirmed hypotheses. Others were educated in disciplines in which theory was viewed as loosely connected hypothetic conjectures. Still others come from educational backgrounds in which little viable theory exists. As a result, the nursing literature contains varying definitions for theory, but this diversity only serves to stimulate further understanding and development of theory.

From our perspective, nursing theory need not be limited to any one theoretic form. A definition that is useful for characterizing nursing theory must be broad enough to include diverse theory types. Our definition of theory is as follows:

> **theory** A creative and rigorous structuring of ideas that project a tentative, purposeful, and systematic view of phenomena.

By our definition, all theory comprises a creative and rigorous structuring of ideas. The ideas are structured as concepts, represented by words as symbols. In order for theory to project a systematic view of phenomena, the concepts contained within the theory must be conveyed as relationship statements and defined within the context of the theory. In theorizing, the theorist creates a language or structure that imparts to theory its systematic nature. Theory is purposive; theorists create theory for some reason. The purpose may take many forms. Theory is tentative and thus is grounded in assumptions, value choices, and the creative and imaginative judgment of the theorist.

Fig. 4-2 summarizes key phrases from the four definitions we have examined. It also shows how these phrases relate to the definition we have synthesized. We show the major characteristics and structural traits of theory that are suggested by our definition of theory. The four definitions we examined were selected to focus on certain characteristics of theory that are con-

Nursing theory: an examination of the concept

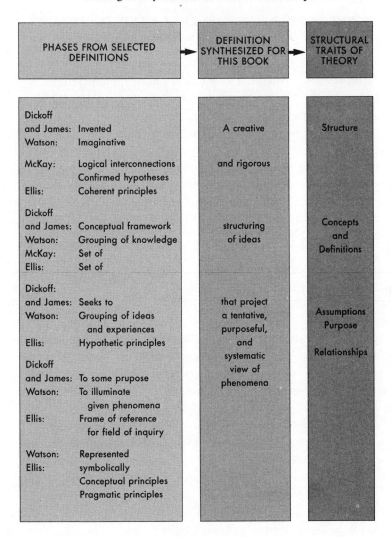

FIG. 4-2

Interrelationships between definitions and features of theory.

sistent with the concept of "theory," but none of the previous definitions address all of those characteristics. The definition we have synthesized incorporates a wide range of methods or forms for the development of theory and represents theory as both process and product. These characteristics of theory provide the basis for determining components used to describe theory that are presented in Chapter 6.

DEFINITIONS OF TERMS RELATED TO THEORY DEVELOPMENT

Once a definition of "theory" is created, it is possible to analyze how theory differs from related terms such as science, philosophy, paradigm, and conceptual framework. Like the word "theory," these terms are highly abstract and have multiple meanings. In order to resolve differences between similar, yet different, terms such as "conceptual framework" and "theory," definitions of both can be created. It is possible to arrive at definitions for different terms that are alike, and it is equally possible that definitions for the same term will reflect fundamental differences in meaning. The definitions of related terms—like our definition of theory—may not be universally accepted, but we believe that they are reasonable and reflect common meanings.

Science. Science is both an approach to the generation of knowledge and the results of using that approach. Science—the process—uses methods that are valid and reliable within a defined area of concern. These methods include different approaches to research, as well as critical and logical thought. Science is also a body of knowledge; that is, it is the facts, theories, and descriptions generated when using empiric processes of science. The processes of science create systematic representations of reality that are accessible to the human senses and are therefore called "empiric." When we use the term "empirics" as a pattern of knowing, we imply that the pattern depends on accessible sensory experience to create knowledge and form understanding. For us, empirics does not require strict adherence to the tenets of traditional science.

Traditional natural science structures empiric knowledge without concern for the intentions of the person or the meaning of behavior. Natural science assumes that the scientist and the object of study are separate and that what is being studied is governed by laws and rules that do not vary. Discovering these laws and rules makes it possible to predict and subsequently control. In this view, the proper procedures of science assume that the scientist's behavior and values do not influence the discovery of knowledge.

Human science approaches draw on the traditions of natural science. These sciences differ in that empiric knowledge development must account for the thinking, feeling, and intentional characteristics of human nature. Because of this, scholars working in the human sciences have begun to develop methods that acknowledge the intimate connection between the scientist and what is studied. These methods are designed to account for the effects of the influence of the scientist on what is studied. The shifts in the assumptions, processes, and outcomes for traditional science that have emerged from the human science perspective are reflected in our approach to theory and knowledge development in nursing. This includes a shift toward understanding rather than prediction, as well as a rejection of the traditional view of control as being neither desirable or possible.

Philosophy. Philosophy is a form of disciplined inquiry for the purpose of discerning general traits of reality. Philosophy is also a body of knowledge about the nature of reality that deals with many phenomena that are not suitable for empiric study. Philosophy contains many branches of thought, each with its own theories. Competing explanations about the nature of reality can exist within the discipline of philosophy. Knowledge development in nursing rests on basic philosophic tenets and assumptions that are derived from selected schools of philosophic thought. Important philosophic foundations that underlie knowledge development include theories about the nature of reality, the nature of knowledge and knowing, and the ways of discerning reality.

Research. Research is application of formalized methods of obtaining reliable and valid knowledge about empiric experience. Research in the human sciences requires multiple processes to generate empiric knowledge and theory. Empiric knowledge gained from research is considered to be repeatable and valid in its conceptions of reality within given limits. Although research is sometimes used to mean a product, as in the phrase, "this is my research," it refers most frequently to the process rather than the outcome.

Fact. A fact is generally held to be an empirically verifiable object, property, or event, meaning that the phenomenon is experienced and named similarly by others. Facts are useful because they reflect common observation on a gross level. If one person observes that "it is raining" and others agree, the statement "it is raining" is accepted as a fact.

Model. A model is a symbolic representation of an empiric experience. The symbolic form of a model may be words, mathematic notations, or physical material, as in a model airplane. One key idea in understanding models is that they are not the real thing, but are an attempt to objectify the concept they represent. A model of any object, property, or event replicates reality with various degrees of precision.

A physical model of some property or event, as well as of an object, is often useful. The properties and events of the physical and biologic world are often modeled to provide a basic understanding of their function. An example is a planetarium, which models the movement of stars and planets in the universe. Modeling human characteristics is difficult, and, when human objects, properties, and events are modeled, the model is less precise because of the complex nature of human characteristics.

It is also possible to model highly abstract concepts. These models consist of such things as words, numbers, letters, or geometric forms. The diagram of the processes for theory development used in this book is an example of a model. Models expressed in language are often called conceptual models, although in one sense all models are conceptual (representative of an idea). Theoretic models are similar to conceptual models but imply less tentativeness. Terms sometimes used interchangeably are "conceptual and theoretic models" and "conceptual and theoretic framework." Within nursing there is considerable overlap among the terms "conceptual model," "conceptual framework," and "theory." For us, conceptual and theoretic models coexist with theory.

Paradigm. The term paradigm implies a world view or ideology, a medium within which the theory, knowledge, and processes for knowing find meaning and coherence and are expressed. A paradigm implies standards or criteria for assigning value or worth to both the processes and products of a discipline, as well as for the methods of knowledge development within a discipline. All of the components of a paradigm are compatible with one another, but wide variation can exist within its structure.

CONCLUSION

In this chapter the difficulty of defining concepts was addressed; four definitions of theory were comparatively analyzed, and a new definition proposed for nursing theory. Definitions of theory-related terms were also discussed, since a full understanding of theory is facilitated by knowledge of its definitions in various contexts. Having established our definition of theory, in Chapter 5 we will examine the processes for generating and developing theory.

Nursing theory: an examination of the concept

REFERENCES

Dickoff J and James P: A theory of theories: a position paper, Nurs Res 17(3):197–203, 1968.

Dickoff J, James P, and Wiedenbach E: Theory in a practice discipline. Part I. Practice-oriented theory, Nurs Res 17(5):415–435, 1968.

Ellis R: Characteristics of significant theories, Nurs Res 17(3):217–222, 1968.

Glaser B and Strauss A: The discovery of grounded theory, Chicago, 1967, Aldine Publishing Co.

Jacox A: Theory construction in nursing: an overview, Nurs Res 23(1):4–13, 1974.

Kaplan A: The conduct of inquiry, New York, 1964, Thomas Y. Crowell Co, Inc.

Levine ME: The four conservation principles of nursing, Nurs Forum, 6(1):45–59, 1967.

McKay RP: Theories, models, and systems for nursing, Nurs Res 18(5):393–399, 1969.

Rogers ME: An introduction to the theoretical basis of nursing, Philadelphia, 1970, FA Davis Co.

Watson J: Nursing: human science and human care, Norwalk, Conn, 1985, Appleton-Century-Crofts.

5

Development of nursing theory

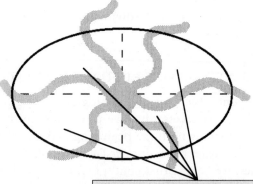

Theory: a creative and rigorous
structuring of ideas that project
a tentative, purposeful, and
systematic view of phenomena.
Chinn and Kramer

There are four processes for creating empiric theory. These
processes include: (1) creating conceptual meaning, (2)
structuring and contextualizing theory, (3) generating and
testing theoretic relationships, and (4) deliberative application
of theory. When all of these processes occur, theory with
practice value evolves.

This chapter presents a description of each of the four processes of theory development: creating conceptual meaning, structuring and contextualizing theory, generating and testing theoretic relationships, and deliberative application of theory. Theory can be developed using any of the processes as a starting point.

Creating conceptual meaning provides a foundation for developing theory. In this chapter we provide a detailed explanation of how conceptual meaning is created, since it is not commonly acknowledged as part of theory development. In addition, we describe the processes of structuring and contextualizing theory, generating and testing theoretic relationships, and deliberative application of theory.

CREATING CONCEPTUAL MEANING

Although creating conceptual meaning is a logical starting point for theory development, it does not necessarily have to be accomplished first. It is a process that can be done by both the beginning and the advanced scholar, and by the novice and expert practitioner (see Chapter 9). As the term for this process implies, we believe that conceptual meaning is something that is created. It does not "exist" as an "out there" reality, but it is deliberately formed from empiric experience. Although this process is critical to all theory development, it is often overlooked as a component of the process (Norris, 1982). Most theorists provide definitions of terms used within theory, but forming word definitions is not the same as creating meaning. Conceptual meaning conveys thoughts, feelings, and ideas that reflect human experience more fully than word definitions.

We have defined the term "concept" as "a complex mental formulation of empiric experience." By "experience" we mean perceptions of the world—objects, other people, visual images, color, movement, sounds, behavior, interactions—the totality of that which is perceived. "Experience" is considered "empiric" when it can be shared and verified by others. How the meaning of a concept forms is depicted in Fig. 5-1. Three sources of experience interact to form the meaning of the idea: (1) the word or other symbolic label, (2) the thing itself (object, property, or event), and (3) feelings, values, and attitudes associated with the word and with the perception of the material thing.

Development of nursing theory

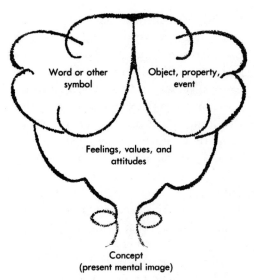

Concept
(present mental image)

FIG. 5-1
The formation of concepts.

Conceptual meaning is created by considering all three sources of expe-riences related to the concept—the *word,* the *thing itself,* and the associated *feelings.* The same word may be used to represent more than one phenome-non. For example, the word symbol "cup" may be used to represent several different kinds of objects or ideas. Each use of the word carries with it dif-ferent perceptions. If the object is a fancy tea cup, a very different mental image forms than if the object is the cup into which a golf ball falls on a putting green. The word symbol "love," a more abstract concept, can be used to describe a feeling toward a parent, child, pet, car, job, or sexual part-ner. A single phenomenon can also be represented by several different words. Each word conveys a slightly different meaning, often nuances that related to socially derived value meanings. For example, the words "automobile," "Chevy," "hot wheels," can all refer to one thing, a car. Using any of these words to describe the object conveys more about the perspective or value of the person using the word than it does about the object itself. The evolution of words and their multiple meanings is complex. Conceptual meaning is created, in part, by increasing our awareness of the range of possible uses and meanings of words. Creating conceptual meaning formulates as exactly as possible what is intended so that misunderstandings about meanings can be avoided.

Feelings, values, and attitudes are inner processes that are associated with empiric experiences and with words. The process of creating conceptual meaning explores the various feelings, attitudes, and values that are associated with the experience and with the word. For example, the word "mother" carries feelings, values, and attitudes that form in human experience with an actual person. Varying experiences with "mother" (the person) account for a range of feelings that different people associate with the word "mother." At the same time, human meaning of the concept "mother" is formed from cultural and societal heritages that all people of a culture share, regardless of individual experiences in early childhood.

Creating conceptual meaning is essentially an empiric approach that depends on mental processes. This means that mental structures, or ideas, are used to represent experience. What is mentally constructed is expressed in words. This process draws on esthetic, ethical, and personal knowing in that mental representations using language depend on creativity that comes from the whole of knowing. The process of creating conceptual meaning assumes common yet unique human experiences and shared meaning among people. At the same time, it is a process that assumes that a person's own subjective construction of reality is more accessible than anything else. This assumption is not traditionally held for methods of science.

Used as an empiric tool in the context of nursing's patterns of knowing, the process of creating conceptual meaning brings dimensions of meaning to a conscious, communicable awareness. Because of the limits of language, the process of creating conceptual meaning also makes it possible to identify the limits of empirics for understanding meaning. Language limitations for expressing meaning lead to discovery and creativity. Language limitations form avenues for self awareness (personal knowing), convey non-empiric dimensions of meaning (esthetic knowing), and suggest value (ethical knowing). The power of language is the power of naming and creating meaning. If a person is told that she is clever, an awareness of self begins to form that may be new to her. At the same time, the word "clever" does not adequately express her rich inner experiences and may not be consistent with her self-knowing. If the word represents a desired value, the description given to her contributes positively to her self awareness. Thus, even though the process of creating conceptual meaning rests primarily on empiric assumptions, the meaning expressed draws on and contributes to the whole of knowing.

There are various methods for creating conceptual meaning. Berthold (1964) described a method for theoretic and empiric clarification of concepts that was closely linked to the tenets and methods of traditional science. Norris (1982) described several different methods for concept clarification. The methods we suggest here arise from our own experience of concept clarification and are informed by the works of Wilson (1963) and Walker and Avant (1988). They are not a "cookbook" approach to achieving a final product. They are exercises, mental gymnastics, and techniques that uncover subtle elements of meaning that can be embedded in concepts. Theories, which are constructed from clarified concepts, help to unravel hidden or difficult nuances of experience that otherwise might remain hidden from view. Methods for creating conceptual meaning are intended to contribute to theory development by strengthening the conceptual quality of theory.

Creating conceptual meaning produces a tentative definition of the concept and a set of tentative criteria for determining if the concept "exists" in a particular situation. We use the word "tentative" because both the definition and the criteria can be revised. The term "tentative" does not mean that "anything goes" or that any definition that suits the author will do. This process is a deliberative, disciplined activity. The person who is creating meaning draws on many sources of data, examines many possible dimensions of meaning, and presents ideas so that they can be tested and challenged in the light of purposes for which the concept is being clarified.

Selecting a concept

An early step in the process of creating conceptual meaning is to select the concept with which to work. An initial concept may change as meanings evolve. Selection begins by identifying a word that communicates an image that approximates the idea you wish to convey. Since what is experienced is not adequately expressed in common language, words may seem quite inadequate at first. You may select a common language word for a concept and eventually assign a specific definition to the word to suit your particular purposes. Or you may borrow a word from another language, combine two or more common words to specify a particular meaning, or make up a phrase or a word. Words that are created to convey a special meaning within a discipline are called "technical" or "professional" terms. These words may only have special meaning within disciplines and have no general or common meaning, or, on the other hand, they may be words that are also used in common language.

Selecting a concept is a process that involves a great deal of ambiguity. You will probably not be satisfied with your early choice of terms to express your ideas. Trying out various alternative words becomes part of the process itself. For example, there is no adequate single term for the idea expressed in the phrase "the use of humans as objects." The term "objectification" is close, but implies some experiences that do not involve the use of humans. The process of working with various terms related to this idea will help to explore various meanings that are possible.

Clarifying your purpose

To provide a sense of direction, you must know why you are creating conceptual meaning. One purpose is to set boundaries or limits so you don't become hopelessly lost in the process. For example, your purpose might be to work with the concept "dependence" for a research project. Eventually you need a clear conceptualization of dependence, as well as ideas about how to measure dependence. Another purpose might be to differentiate between two closely related concepts such as "sympathy" and "empathy." In this case your concern is to create definitions that do this, based on thorough familiarity with meanings that are possible.

Another reason for creating conceptual meaning is to examine the ways in which concepts are used in existing writings. The concept of intuition, for example, frequently appears in nursing literature, but with diverse meanings. The meanings conveyed reflect different assumptions about the phenomena. As you become aware of these meanings, you can explore the extent to which the meanings are consistent with your own view.

Other purposes for creating conceptual meaning include generating research hypotheses, formulating nursing diagnoses, or simply practicing the process. Whatever your purpose, clarifying it can provide a sense of direction when you seem to be hopelessly lost.

Data sources

Once a concept has been selected, the process of creating conceptual meaning proceeds by using multiple data sources to generate and refine criteria that include indicators for the concept. The sources of data you choose and the extent to which you use various sources depends on your purposes.

Definitions. One source of data that provides information about conceptual meaning are definitions and word usages of the concept you are exploring. Existing definitions are often circular and will not give a complete sense of meaning for the concept, but they do help to clarify common ideas and uses. Existing definitions help to identify common or core elements about objects, perceptions, or feelings that can be represented by the word. They are also useful to trace the origin of words that give clues to core meaning.

Dictionary definitions provide synonyms and antonyms and convey commonly accepted ways in which words are used. They are not designed to explain the full range of perceptions associated with a word, particularly when the word has a unique use with a discipline or represents a relatively abstract concept.

Existing theories provide a source of definitions that sometimes extend beyond the limits of common linguistic usage. Theoretic definitions and ways in which concepts are used in the context of the theory convey meanings that pertain to the domain of the discipline from which the theory comes.

The term "mother" as defined in the dictionary, for example, refers to the social and biologic role of parenting and includes a few characteristics of the role such as authority and affection. In the context of psychologic theories, the meanings conveyed with respect to the values, roles, functions, and characters of people who are mothers are almost endless and include attachment, guilt, responsibility, power, and powerlessness.

Cases. Another useful approach to creating conceptual meaning is constructing cases that represent the experience you are exploring. This involves presenting an object or instance of the experience or constructing a scenario that illustrates the experience. From these cases you can identify and reflect on criteria for the concept.

Model cases. One type of case is a model case. In constructing a model case you describe or present an instance of an experience so that "If this is not X, then nothing is." This represents the concept to the best of your present understanding. For concrete concepts such as "cup," a model case is relatively easy. An ordinary teacup, for example, can be presented for everyone to see and hold. The people who examine the object can then verify, "If this is not a cup, then nothing is." To demonstrate the concept "red" (a property), a model case is more difficult. You can physically present to the group something that you perceive as red in color and find out if they agree that this is what "red" is. The model case would be the color sample that most often is perceived as "red" by other people.

When you deal with highly abstract concepts, the task of constructing model cases is more difficult. Usually model cases of abstract concepts involve experiences and circumstances that are described in words. For a concept such as "mothering," your model case might begin with an event: an infant cries, and an adult picks up the infant. The event is a start, but your observers might object, saying that this description represents only the physical act of "picking up " and is not necessarily "mothering." Your model case develops until there is enough substance so that people respond to the case by forming a mental image of "mothering." As you build on the scenario of an adult picking up an infant to represent "mothering," you could include various circumstances, behaviors, motives, attitudes, and feelings that surround the act of picking up the infant. You paint a picture, or tell a story, so that people can confirm that this indeed is "mothering." As this and other model cases are created, you can compare various meanings in the experience and define commonalities and differences.

It is often useful to alternatively include and exclude various features of model cases in order to reflect on how central each feature is to the meaning you are creating. For example, in the model case of "mothering," the adult might initially be portrayed to be female. Later you might portray a male adult in the same case. In the absence of any evidence one way or the other, you might tentatively decide that the idea of "mothering" you are creating will be deliberately limited to instances involving female adults. Since your decision is tentative, you can change your construction for another purpose or circumstance. You can acknowledge the "fact" that some males "mother," but for your purpose your idea deliberately includes the characteristic of female adults.

While you are working with model cases, pose the question "What is it that makes this an instance of this concept?" The responses to this question form the basis for a tentative list of criteria. In early stages the criteria may be quite detailed and may be the essential characteristics associated with the concept, given the meanings you deliberately decide to include. The criteria are designed to make it possible to recognize the concept when it occurs empirically and to differentiate this concept from other related concepts. For example, in the case of "mothering," you would want to be able to recognize mothering when it happens, as well as to distinguish mothering from such related phenomena as "caring," "nurturing," or "helping."

Impressions regarding the criteria begin to form as you design model cases. As you work with various possible features of the model cases, you begin to form ideas about which features are essential and why, as well as their qualitative features. These ideas become the criteria for the concept.

Contrary cases. Contrary cases are those that are certainly *not* an instance of the concept. These may be similar in some respects, but they represent something that most observers would recognize easily as what you are *not* talking about. For concrete concepts, contrary cases are relatively easy. A saucer or a spoon can be presented, and most observers in Western cultures would agree that these things are not cups. A spoon may hold liquids that people sip from, but it would not be a cup. A saucer that a cup sits on would also clearly not be a cup. A contrary case for the color red might be the color green. For the concept of restlessness a case portraying calmness could be presented as a contrary case.

As you consider contrary cases, ask: "What makes this instance different from the concept that was selected?" By comparing the differences between model and contrary cases, you will begin to revise the model cases. In turn, you can also revise, add to, or delete from the tentative list of criteria that are emerging. For example, one of the traits that distinguishes a cup from a saucer or a spoon is the shape of the cup. You might already discern that this is an essential feature by looking only at the cup. But, when you see the spoon and saucer, the shape stands out in sharp contrast, and your description of essential features of the shape of the cup can be more complete and precise. As you compare the objects, you may also decide that the volume of liquid that a cup holds is an important distinguishing characteristic. Later, when you consider miniature tea cups as cases, you might decide that volume is not an essential quality, especially if your other criteria are sufficient to distinguish which objects can be called a cup for your purpose.

Related cases. Related cases are instances that represent a different but similar concept. A different word is generally used to label these instances, but the experience has several features in common with the one you have selected for study. When you consider related cases, your ideas become much clearer about the meanings that are central to the concept you are exploring.

In the case of a "cup" you might consider a drinking glass. For the concept of "red" you might consider a red-orange hue and a magenta. For the concept of "mothering," you could design a case of "tending" that would be similar to the model case. You might make a child care worker the adult person, or substitute an elderly person for the infant. Again you consider differences and similarities between the model and related cases, and revise the tentative criteria to reflect your new insights.

Borderline cases. A borderline case is an instance of metaphoric or pseudo applications of the word. The same word is generally used for these instances, but the actual experience is usually quite different from the one you have selected for study. Poetry and lyrics to music provide rich sources of metaphoric uses of words. In the evolution of language, the metaphoric meanings of words carry powerful messages that often persist as new usages emerge and thus illuminate core meaning. The metaphoric meanings for the concept of "red" are an excellent example. "Red" as a word and as a color has become a symbol for communism. The metaphoric messages in this usage symbolize human experiences of blood, violence, passion, loss. To give a "cup of cheer" is an exemplary borderline usage of the term "cup." This highlights the feature of cups as capable of holding something.

For the concept of "mothering," a borderline case may be a description of an adult bird caring for newly hatched chicks. You might use this case to help clarify whether a motive to care is necessary for your meaning. Ask what happens to your meaning if you perceive of mothering as something that happens by "instinct."

You will probably invent other varieties of cases in the process of creating conceptual meaning. How cases are classified is not critical. Their important function is to assist you to discern the full range of possible meaning, so that you can design a meaning that is useful for your purpose.

Visual images. Visual images that already exist such as photographs, cartoons, calendars, paintings, and drawings are useful data sources in concept clarification. It may also be important for you to deliberately create images that represent the concept being clarified rather than use existing sources. Whether you personally create and examine an image or ask others to create images, the idea is to compare them for similarities and differences. Advertisements and photographs documenting the concept "depression," for example, provide information about conceptual meaning. Often visual imagery will highlight some aspect of the concept that is significant. On other occasions visual imagery may raise questions about the essential nature of the phenomena that are important to refining criteria. Visual images that represent concepts very well also highlight difficulties in expressing meaning linguistically. A photograph may express the concept of dignity, yet the essence of dignity expressed by the photo is impossible to describe.

Popular and classical literature. A variety of literature resources can provide information about conceptual meaning. Whereas cases evolve from your personal experience, the literature reflects meanings arising from the experiences of others. Classical prose and poetry are often rich sources of meaning for concepts used in nursing. For example, images of love and longing may be found in the poetic works of Emily Dickinson. Louisa May Alcott's classic story, *Little Women,* provides information about the nature of intimacy and caring. The popular current literature is also a source of valuable data about conceptual meaning. Popular self-help books on such topics as stress management and codependency can enrich conceptual data. Fairy tales, myths, fables, and stories provide relevant data, depending on the concept you are exploring. Usages for words that are expressed in popular jargon and cartoons may highlight borderline meaning. For example, when a 5-year-old jumps up and down and exclaims, "I'm so *anxious* for my birthday to be here!", the meaning of "anxious" is not the same meaning for anxiety that concerns nurses. What the nursing usage conveys is the physical agitation that accompanies the experience of anxiety within the context of nursing practice.

Music. The imagery of music may be useful in concept clarification. Music can effectively convey the rhythms and balance inherent in many life events with which nurses deal. Cecile Chaminade's *Concertino for Flute and Orchestra,* for example, involves cadences and dynamics that can be said to reflect both passion and playfulness.

Professional literature. Meanings for concepts can be explored from within the context of professional literature. This literature often provides meanings that are pertinent to the practice of nursing. For example, philosophers, as well as nurses, have written about the concept of "presence" as a way of being with another. Both are valuable sources for exploring meanings. When the literature of other disciplines is considered, meanings may not clearly apply to nursing, but meaning found across disciplines contributes to concept clarification.

People sources. Peers, coworkers, hospitalized persons, and professional workers who are not nurses can provide valuable information about the meaning of a concept. It may be useful to seek the opinions of others about the meaning a concept has, particularly if your direct experience with the concept is limited. Nurses who work with the concept daily may be able to shed light on nuances of meaning that will markedly affect how meaning is integrated into theory. For example, a nurse who works with people whose lung function is severely compromised might observe that anxiety, although usually characterized by increased activity, evokes a different reaction. Rather than random activity, it may be accompanied by a deliberate quieting of behavior to conserve energy.

As you can surmise, the sources of data that can be used in concept clarification are potentially inexhaustible. Undoubtedly you will think of others that are useful to you as you work on clarifying concepts. What sources to use and how to use them unfolds as the process of concept clarification creates conceptual meaning.

Exploring contexts and values

Social contexts within which experience and the values that grow out of experience occur form important cultural meanings that influence mental representations of that experience. Consider, for example, the concept of "judgment" if you are a student taking an examination, a realtor assessing a home for sale, a person scoring a gymnastics meet, or a magistrate preparing to levy a sentence. When you explore the various meanings acquired by virtue of the context, you will probably become aware of meanings you had not previously considered.

One way to imagine various contexts is to place your model cases in different contexts and ask, "What next?" You mentally imagine the practical outcomes of your conceptual meaning in its context. For example, if you place your model case of the color red in the context of a magazine advertisement, what symbolic meaning is conveyed? What advertising results does the advertiser intend? If the color red is placed in the context of traffic signs and symbols, what meaning does the color now convey? What behavioral responses do you now expect? As you consider various possible combinations of context, you will clarify how meanings are influenced by the context.

Values are also revealed by placing the concept in a subtly differing context. For example, you might consider mothering in the context of an elementary school classroom. The concept of "mothering" has a relatively positive connotation for most people. Most people agree that humans need "good" mothering to grow and develop adequately. But people differ widely in what they consider to be "good" mothering; these differences often have to do with the cultural context. For example, there would probably be considerable disagreement as to whether what happens in a schoolroom is "mothering." What is considered mothering reflects deeply embedded cultural values. When you consider your model case placed in several different social contexts, you create an avenue for perceiving important values and make deliberate choices concerning them.

Formulating criteria

Criteria for the concept emerge gradually as you consider definitions, various cases, other data sources, and context and values. Criteria are always tentative, but they provide guidelines for recognizing the empiric experience you want to represent and for differentiating it from other similar instances.

As you develop the criteria, you will naturally refine them so that they reflect the meaning you intend. Criteria should express both qualitative and quantitative aspects of meaning and should suggest a definition of the word. Since criteria are more complex than a word definition, they amplify this meaning and suggest direction for the processes of developing theory.

To illustrate the function of criteria for a concept, consider how you might convey the idea of one U.S. dollar in coins to a person who is not familiar with American money. One way is to present all possible combinations of coins to the individual, who then memorizes the combinations in order to consistently collect the right coins together to yield an equivalent of $1. Another approach is to provide guidelines to assist the individual to recognize and compose the various combinations independently. A model case might be presented using three quarters, one dime, two nickels, and five pennies. Realizing many other combinations are possible, criteria are created from the model case to cover all other possible combinations. The model case is chosen deliberately to include all the types of coins available, so that in examining the case several characteristics of all possibilities emerge. One feature is that the units of the various coins used add up to an equivalent of 100 pennies—the smallest possible coin value. However, this criterion alone may not be sufficient for someone who is not familiar with the monetary system being used; thus other criteria are created to ensure that all other possible combinations are recognized. You might consider the weight of the possible coin combinations, the colors of the coins, and their metallic makeup, as well as the exchange value of each coin. All of these features may be used, but criteria should convey, as simply as possible, the information needed by a novice to collect one U.S. dollar in coins. The facts that any color combination or any number of coins up to 100 may be used as criteria. A criterion involving metallic content of the coins might serve as an adequate criterion and may even be the most precise of all possible criteria. But if your purpose is to assist a person from another country to understand how to make a dollar out of change, you would not select the metallic content as a criterion because it is impractical for that purpose.

For concrete objects criteria may be relatively simple. For the concept of "cup," examples of criteria may be as follows:
1. The object is cylindric or conical in shape, with one closed and one open end.
2. The object is capable of containing physical matter.
3. The height is between 3 and 7 inches, and the widest diameter is 3 to 4 inches.
4. When the object contains liquid, it must be capable of safely holding hot liquids.

Notice that this set of criteria is phrased so that "styrofoam cup" and "golfing green cup" can be included. This choice is guided by the purpose. If you needed to make sure that the golfing green cup was not included as a "cup," you might revise the criteria to include: "the object is capable of being held in the hand, regardless of what it contains." This criterion places a limit on the volume and weight of the cup and implies that it must be a portable object.

Developing criteria for more abstract concepts is a more complex process, and the criteria are often more abstract. Criteria for the concept of "mothering" might be:
1. Visual contact must be observed to be directed from the mothering person to the person who receives mothering.
2. The person who receives mothering must be physically touched by the mothering person.
3. Some positive feeling must be experienced by the mothering person and by the person who receives mothering.

4. There must be a reciprocal interaction between the two people.

5. Vocalization by the mothering person must occur.

These criteria do not limit the mothering person by gender, age, or species. The "mother" could be an elderly, male bird! Nor do the criteria specify that the person who receives mothering is an infant. If the purpose of applying the criteria is to distinguish between instances of "mothering" and "fathering," these criteria would need to be revised to at least specify gender. If the purpose were to differentiate between "mothering" and "neglect," they might be adequate.

A frequent question that arises in the course of concept clarification is: "How do I know that the meaning I have created is right?" In the context of concept clarification, it is not useful to think in terms of right or wrong. It *is* important to consider whether the meaning you have created reflects a reasonable meaning, was carefully derived, and is useful for your purposes. If your aims reflect valued nursing goals, if you have been careful in choosing and using resources, and if you understand why you have made the choices you have, you will have created a useful meaning. Additional processes for theory development will provide a "check" on conceptual meaning and will help refine and illuminate whether the meaning created is valuable.

Conceptual meaning and problems of theoretic development

Problems associated with conceptual meaning often underlie other problems involved in developing theory. A major challenge with respect to generating and testing theoretic relationships is the selection of empiric indicators for a concept. When research reports give conflicting results, the differences are sometimes tied to the use of different definitions and empiric indicators for the concept. If you explore the conceptual meanings within research reports, you can often clarify the extent to which differing conceptual meanings account for the differing research findings. As you carry out the processes for creating conceptual meaning, you will be able to suggest a full range of possible empiric indicators for a concept. You will also be able to identify the limits of empiric approaches in specifying indicators for a phenomenon.

Consider, for example, the concept of "mothering" and the sample criteria we gave in the previous section. These criteria include characteristics that can be observed empirically. They are "reciprocal interaction," "visualization," "touch," and "vocalization." The criterion that states that "some positive feeling must be experienced by the mothering person and the person who receives mothering" might be one of the most important distinguishing features of your intended meaning for "mothering"; but it does not lend itself to objective observation. It can be assessed indirectly by asking mothers to describe their feelings.

Conceptual meaning is fundamental if you must distinguish one concept from another closely related one. This is often the case when you are generating and testing relationships or structuring and contextualizing theory. The processes of creating conceptual meaning make it possible to propose differentiating features that guide research and theory structuring activities. Consider the concepts of "tending" and "mothering." Individuals tend to the needs of others in many different contexts, and mothers tend children. A question to be resolved might be: "Is there a particular kind of 'tending' that occurs with 'mothering'?" You can examine a related case of a sitter tending children to determine if any characteristic of "tending" is within your idea of "mothering." As you explore various differentiating features of the central concept, your ideas will become clearer, and the structure of your theory or research study will improve. Concept clarification helps to make decisions about the qualitative dimensions of criteria such as whether they always need to be evident or if they may be expressed with different intensities. For example, you may decide that, for the concept of mothering, the expression of positive feeling *must* be present, but the degree to which it occurs may vary.

In creating conceptual meaning, the challenge is to evolve a useful and adequate meaning from among a range of possibilities. Although case techniques that are associated with creating conceptual meaning are very useful, when they are supplemented with other data sources, a richer meaning for concepts evolves.

STRUCTURING AND CONTEXTUALIZING THEORY

Structuring and contextualizing theory involves forming systematic linkages between and among concepts, resulting in a formal theoretic structure. There are many approaches that can be used (Dubin, 1978; Newman, 1979; Reynolds, 1971; Walker and Avant, 1988). The choice of a particular approach depends on your purposes for developing the theory, what you already know or assume to be "true," and your underlying philosophic ideas about the nature of nursing knowledge. If you begin with an entirely new idea about something and with very little reported about it in the existing literature, the form of the theory that you construct may be a categorization of the concepts into a relational taxonomy that essentially describes your ideas. If you begin with an idea that builds on other theorists' descriptions, you might develop a theoretic structure that provides explanations of complex interrelationships between concepts. If you are structuring theory as an outcome of grounded research, the interrelationships between data clusters guide the structure you create for the theory.

Approaches to structuring and contextualizing theory include:
- *Identifying and defining the concepts.* Identifying and defining concepts specify the ideas on which the theoretic structure is built. Definitions can be composed using the processes for creating conceptual meaning, or they can be borrowed from other theories or formulated from multiple other sources. They should identify as clearly and concisely as possible the theoretic meaning of important terms within the theory.
- *Identifying assumptions.* Identifying assumptions clarifies the basic underlying "truths" from which and within which theoretic reasoning proceeds.
- *Clarifying the context within which the theory is placed.* Contextual placement describes the circumstances within which the theoretic relationships are expected to be empirically relevant. Clear statements regarding context are particularly important if the theory is to be applied in practice.
- *Designing relationship statements.* Designing theoretic statements describes the projected and evolving relationships between and among the concepts of the theory. These statements, taken as a whole, provide the substance and the form of the theory.

Identifying and defining concepts

Structuring theory requires that you identify the concepts that will form the theory. The concepts can come from life experiences, clinical practice, basic or applied research, knowledge of the literature, and from the formal processes of creating conceptual meaning. Often theory emerges because of a conviction that existing knowledge and theories are not adequate to represent an experience.

Some types of concepts are better suited for theory development than others. Concepts that are extremely abstract carry broad meanings and refer to a wide range of empiric experience. These are usually not suitable as a beginning point for theory development. Concepts such as "social structure," "politics," or "love," for example, refer to such a broad range of empiric experience that defining them within the limits of empiric inquiry is extremely difficult. Such concepts, however, can be useful in considering the context within which the theory is placed. If concepts are extremely narrow and concrete, they refer to only a narrow range of experiences, and the level of abstraction may not be sufficient for theoretic purposes. For example, concepts such as "toothache," "menstrual pain," or "backache" apply to relatively few instances of "pain." "Pain" is a more suitable concept from which to develop theory.

As the concepts are specified or begin to form, early ideas about the structure of their relationships begin to emerge. There are usually one or two primary or central concepts around which the theoretic relationships build. Thinking about possible relationships helps to clarify what concepts the theory needs to include. Previous research, existing theories, philosophies, and personal experience provide a background for forming theoretic relationships. Initially you might simply note concepts that you think are related on the basis of your experience, what you find in the literature, or ongoing research.

An assumption that is inherent in most empiric theory is the concept of linear time. If your emerging theory is to be predictive, this structure influences the type and substance of the concepts required for the theory. Antecedent, coincident or intervening, and consequent concepts imply prediction within a linear time frame. Antecedent concepts are those experiences that you identify as coming before other concepts. Coincident concepts are those that coexist in time. Intervening concepts are also coincident and have a particular influence on relationships among concepts that are specified in the theory. Consequent concepts are those that follow another.

Some theories place antecedents in a "causal" relationship with those that follow. Other theories rest on a philosophic view that rejects the idea of causation. Instead, the ideas of influence or effect are used to explain relationships over time. If a primary concept within your developing theory is stress, you might propose that previous childhood experiences "cause" the stress experience, or you might consider childhood experience as an antecedent that influences the stress experience.

Consequents can also imply causation. For example, once a person experiences "stress," consequents of that experience can be thought of as happening as a result of the stress. Changes in mental functioning, changes in sleep and rest patterns, and changes in relationships with other people might be theoretic concepts structured to reflect phenomena "caused" by the stress.

The idea of intervening concepts can be used to shift from a view of causation to one of influence. Intervening concepts are those that influence the relationships between antecedent experiences, the event itself, and its consequents. For example, the central concept of stress might be viewed as being influenced by the antecedent experiences of childhood, and sleep patterns might be viewed as an intervening variable that influences the relationship between the childhood experience and present stress.

As initial ideas are formed concerning relationships between concepts, the concepts themselves become clearer. Some concepts might be grouped together and assigned more abstract terms to comprise a new concept. This occurs especially when theory is structured using inductive theory development processes such as grounded theory. For example, you might begin to see that "time of day" and "season of year" could be grouped to become components of the more abstract concept "biologic rhythms."

As the concepts of the theory are identified and conceptualized, theoretic definitions emerge. Theoretic definitions form the basis for and reflect empiric indicators and operational definitions for concepts that are needed for research. Theoretic definitions convey the general meaning of the concept. Operational definitions are different from theoretic definitions in that they indicate as exactly as possible how the concept is to be assessed in a specific study (see pp. 100 to 101). For example, a theoretic definition for the concept of "mothering" might read:

mothering An interaction between a human adult and child that conveys reciprocal feelings of attachment. The interaction is behaviorally expressed by reciprocal visual contact, touching, and vocalization.

This theoretic definition gives a general idea of empiric indicators for the concept, which in turn imply operational definitions. The first part of the definition provides a general meaning for the term. The second part suggests behaviors associated with the concept that can be assessed.

Notice that the theoretic definition is consistent with tentative criteria for the concept "mothering" (see p. 91), but the definition serves a different purpose from the criteria. The criteria are specific and useful as a foundation for construction of theory and for empiric study of the concept. The theoretic definition summarizes the insights that are formed in creating conceptual meaning and concisely conveys the essential meaning of the concept.

Identifying assumptions

Assumptions are underlying "givens" that are presumed to be true. They are not intended to be empirically tested, but they can be challenged philosophically and may be investigated empirically. Philosophic assumptions form the philosophic grounding for a theory; if they are challenged, the substance of the entire theory is also challenged on philosophic grounds. Nonphilosophic assumptions (that is, assumptions that could be empirically investigated but aren't within the context of the theory) also affect the value of the entire theory. Stated assumptions are easy to recognize, but many assumptions are implied, or not stated, and are difficult to recognize. An example of an underlying assumption that is usually not stated is: "Human beings are complex." For theories that involve human experience this statement can be taken as reasonably "true." However, many commonly accepted "truths" about human existence gain new significance within a theoretic context, and they need to be stated even if they seem self-evident. For example, if a theory were to include the concept "death," certain underlying assumptions about the nature of life and death would influence the essential ideas of the theory, and these need to be stated. A theory that is based on the view of death as a transition to another form of life will be very different from a theory that views death as the end of life.

Rogers (1970) made her assumption explicit that human beings are unified wholes possessing their own integrity and manifesting characteristics that are more than and different from the sum of their parts. On the surface, this seems to be a perfectly reasonable and sensible statement, but it is significant because it is an assumption that is not common to all nursing theory. As an assumption, it does not require empiric evidence, but it is fundamental to the relationship statements she proposed, and the relationships are empirically tested.

Assumptions influence all aspects of structuring and contextualizing theory. If the assumption "holism" is used as a basis for a theory of "mothering," interrelated concepts must be consistent with a holistic view of human experience. Patterns of behavior that reflect the whole would be reflected in the theoretic concepts. These might include patterns of movement and communication. In contrast, if human beings were assumed to be biologic and social organisms, the concepts of a mothering theory might include such concepts as physical responses and cultural mores.

Clarifying the context

Theoretic relationships must be placed within a context if the theory is to be useful for practice. If a theory of "mothering" is meant to apply only to the interactions of women and children in Western cultures, these limits on the applicability of the theory must be stated. As the theory is extended, it might be found to be useful for other cultures and for other kinds of intimate relationships such as adult-child, adult-adult, or adult-animal interactions. Theory that arises from inductive methods is contextualized as a result of the process itself.

Contexts that are very broad or very narrow limit the applicability of theory. A theory that is cognitively structured as an explanation for all cultures will probably not be useful for any culture. Conversely, a theory that is structured within the context of a single institution (for example, one hospital) will probably not be useful for other settings.

Designing relationship statements

Relationship statements describe, explain, or predict the nature of the interactions between the concepts of the theory. The statements range from those that simply relate two concepts to relatively complex statements that account for interactions among three or more concepts. Theories usually contain several levels of relationship statements, which comprise a reasonably complete explanation of how the concepts of the theory interact. The relationships begin to take form as the concepts are identified and emerge, but the process of designing the relationship statements requires specific attention to the substance, direction, strength, and quality of interactions between concepts.

Consider a relationship statement that might be formulated using the concept of "mothering." A theorist might propose that, as an adult's visual contact with an infant increases, the infant's visual contact with the adult will also increase. This relationship statement speculates that one event (increased adult visual contact) precedes a second event (increased infant visual contact). This relationship also describes a substantive interaction (visual contact) as a component of mothering. It implies direction (increase) as part of the interaction.

A more complex relational statement addresses further dimensions of quality, contexts, and circumstances that are proposed. Such a statement might take the form:

Under the conditions of C1 . . . Cn, if X occurs, then Y will occur.

Or, to use the illustration involving the concept of "mothering":

When an adult mothering figure and an infant are in close proximity (C1),

and

when the adult has a negative feeling toward the infant (C2),

and

when the frequency of physical contact is limited (C3),

then,

if the adult's frequency of visual contact decreases, the infant's frequency of visual contact will also decrease.

A relationship may also be designed to introduce new concepts to the potential theory. Initially such a relationship might read:

If the infant's frequency of visual contact is not sufficient to satisfy the mother, the adult's frequency of visual contact will increase in a conscious effort to engage the infant in interaction.

This introduces the concept of "awareness" and an alternate value, not simply positive or negative, for the concept "visual contact." That alternate value is "sufficient to satisfy," which is not empirically observable. As the theory is developed further, possible empiric indicators for "satisfaction" might be created. Or this dimension of the theory might be viewed as something beyond the realm of empirics. In this way the theory not only stimulates the creation of new empiric knowledge, but also opens possibilities for exploring and integrating other ways of knowing. Although empiric theory is primarily designed to propose and create empiric relationships, it can also contain concepts and relationships that integrate ethical, esthetic, and personal knowing.

GENERATING AND TESTING THEORETIC RELATIONSHIPS

Generating and testing theoretic relationships involves a focus on the correspondence of the ideas of the theory with empiric experience (Dubin, 1978; Newman, 1979; Reynolds, 1971; Glaser and Strauss, 1967). Since theories are abstractions of reality, a translation is made from the theoretic to the empiric (deductive approach) and from the empiric to the theoretic (inductive approach). A theory cannot be "proven," but it is possible to gather empiric support for a theory. If the evidence does not support or create theoretic relationships, the ideas of the theory cannot be sustained as theory. Alternative theoretic explanations are then considered, based on the empiric evidence.

The activity of generating and testing theoretic relationships draws on one or more subcomponents: (1) empirically grounding emerging relationships, (2) explicating empiric indicators, and (3) validating relationships through empiric methods.

Empirically grounding emerging relationships

The process of empirically grounding emerging relationships involves connecting experiences with representations of those experiences. When an abstract theoretic relationship is taken as the starting point, the theorist presents empiric evidence that suggests empiric support for the projected relationship. This is usually presented as examples within the narrative explanations of the theory. When this process is taken as the starting point, the theorist selects a social context in which the phenomenon under consideration is likely to be observed and observes the interactions and circumstances of that context. From the observations, the theorist derives relationship statements that are "grounded" in empiric evidence, a process called grounded theory (Glaser and Strauss, 1967). A variety of inductive approaches can also be used to ground emerging relationships. Inductive grounding of emerging relationships gradually evolves into a theoretic structure that can, in turn, form the basis for deducing relationships.

Explicating empiric indicators

Empiric indicators and operational definitions are used to represent concepts as variables in empiric research and are empirically formed for concepts arising from inductive approaches. Formally structured theory can propose empiric indicators, but, until these are put into operation in research, they remain speculative. Using the ideas in actual research makes it possible to refine the ideas of the theory.

Consider the following abstract relationship statement:

As the adult's eye contact increases, the infant's eye contact will increase.

A research project is designed to obtain empiric evidence concerning the use of "eye contact" as an empiric indicator of "mothering." Details such as length of gaze and frequency of eye contact are specified for the relatively abstract concept of "eye contact." In order to use these indicators, the researcher creates a method for observing and timing the length of gaze and the frequency of eye contact.

Part of the process for identifying empiric indicators, especially when primarily deductive processes are used, is to state operational definitions. Operational definitions specify the standards or criteria to be used in making the observations. For example, an operational definition of the term "gaze" might be "a steady, direct, visual focusing on an object that lasts at least 3 seconds." This definition indicates what "gaze" is (the empiric indicator for "visual contact"), characteristics that are to used in calling a behavior a "gaze" (direct visual focusing on an object), and a standard time parameter that distinguishes "gaze" from other related behaviors such as "glance" or "look."

It is more difficult to refine empiric indicators for concepts that are more abstract than the concept "eye contact." Many concepts related to nursing (for example, anxiety, body image, or self-esteem) are highly abstract and cannot be directly measured. Tests and tools have been constructed to provide an indirect estimate of traits such as these. The fact that they cannot be measured directly does not mean they are nonexistent or cannot be assessed. The empiric challenge is to refine ideas about and evidence for empiric indicators so that estimates of relationships can be explored. The difficulties inherent in such situations can be compared to trying to describe what a tomato tastes like. Once a person bites a tomato, that person "knows" how it tastes. The descriptions of that taste are not at all adequate in comparison to the actual taste experience. Descriptions of concepts like anxiety also fall short of the actual human experience. However, if the concept is important for nursing, even a limited study of the experience can be useful.

One approach that can be used to derive empiric measures for abstract nursing concepts is to use multiple empiric indicators to form operational definitions. For example, anxiety might be measured using a self-report tool. The tool can be constructed to include many sensations that are generally indicative of anxiety. The operational definition of the concept "anxiety" then becomes what is assessed with the use of the tool. Anxiety might also be empirically assessed by observing a person's behavior and the physiologic indicators of adrenocortical function. The operational definitions would include specific ways to "measure" the behaviors observed and the specific range of laboratory test results associated with "anxiety." All of these empiric indicators are possible. If they are used together in situations in which the experience of anxiety is likely to occur, the study will provide substantive evidence about the usefulness of each measure as an empiric indicator.

When inductive research processes form the basis for refining empiric indicators, the indicators are directly or indirectly "observed" and are used to form concepts. Determining empiric indicators for concepts becomes important when inductively generated empiric concepts are deductively tested and extended into other contexts.

Validating relationships through empiric methods

Generating and testing theoretic relationships also requires creating a design that "tests" designated relationships. Designs may be proposed after theory is structured (deductive) or may generate theory that, because of the design, is considered to be "tested." Systematic research designs that deductively test specific relationships incorporate several features. One is that the design provides a means to ensure that the proposed relationship is actually the one that accounts for the study findings. For example, if a study concludes that a mother's gaze prompts an infant's gaze in return, the researcher needs to consider ways to be sure that it is actually the mother's gaze that accounts for the infant's behavior. Typically the researcher designs the study so that other factors that could influence the behavior of the infants in the study (for example, sensory experiences that might affect the process of visual interaction such as noise, touch, or visual distractions) are held constant, or accounted for. The purpose of deductively testing any relationship statement is to provide empiric evidence that the relationships proposed in the theory are adequate when represented in a specific situation. With each approach to design that is used, the research question or hypothesis is revised to suit the type of design selected. Empiric evidence based on many different approaches to research design provides a basis for judging the adequacy of the theory. If theoretic statements are deductively tested and not supported by empiric evidence, one or more of four possibilities can account for the disparity between the theory and empiric findings:

1. *The concepts are faulty.* The process of creating conceptual meaning can be used to determine if the definitions and meanings of the concepts under study are clear and if they are well differentiated from other related concepts. If they are not, theoretic revisions can be made, resulting in new approaches to empiric study.

2. *The relationship statement is faulty.* The processes of theory structuring and contextualizing can be used to examine the logic or form of the statements. Given the benefit of the empiric evidence, new insights regarding the form and structure of the theory might emerge. The theorist can revise the theoretic relationship statements on the basis of these insights.

3. *The empiric indicators for the concept are faulty.* The empiric evidence might point to new possibilities for empiric indicators or suggest revisions in the existing indicators. This process is particularly important when the empiric indicators represent highly abstract concepts and are constructed out of speculative ideas about how the concepts can be observed empirically.

4. *The operational definitions are faulty.* Typically, conflicting research results are attributed to faulty operational definitions and the related measurement problems of empiric research. This is a possibility, but accurate measurement depends on adequately conceived concepts, sound theoretic statements, and adequate empiric indicators. If these are all in place, it is then reasonable to consider problems in operationalization.

When inductive methods are used to generate theoretic relationships, the relationships may be considered valid if processes for generating them are carefully done. When relationships are deduced from inductively generated theory, they can be tested. When this occurs, any problems with faulty concepts, relational statements, empiric indicators, and operational definitions will become evident.

DELIBERATIVE APPLICATION OF THEORY

Deliberative application of theory draws on research methods to ensure that the theory can be applied in practice to achieve practice goals. The theoretic relationships are systematically examined in the practice setting, and the results are recorded and assessed to determine how well the theory "works" to achieve the desired outcomes. Testing of theoretic relationships may also occur in the clinical setting, but, when this occurs, the setting is usually altered in order to focus on the nature of the theoretic relationship. Inductive methods that generate theoretic relationships may evolve from nonpractice settings. The extent to which the theory "works" in practice settings needs to be assessed. Deliberative application of theory shifts the focus from testing and generating relationships to gathering evidence as to how the clinical setting itself is affected by the application of the theory. The question shifts away from the soundness of the theoretic relationships to questions concerning the value of the theory in relation to the goals of nursing.

For example, you might be developing a theory concerning the alleviation of pain. The theory generated from an inductive process and empiric evidence testing the theoretic relationships supports the developing theory. Deliberative application involves using the theory in practice and studying the effect of its use on the quality of life, the quality of nursing care, or the processes of health.

Deliberative application of theory has three subcomponents. These are: (1) selecting the clinical setting, (2) determining outcome variables for practice, and (3) implementing a method of study.

Selecting the clinical setting

The clinical setting for deliberative application can be any setting in which nursing is practiced in which the theoretic relationships can be observed. Some phenomena such as the experience of powerlessness, alienation, or separation tend to occur in hospitals or other traditional care settings. Other phenomena such as decision-making are common to a wide variety of settings such as homes, workplaces, hospitals, and community centers. The setting is selected in part because the theory under study is perceived to be useful for that setting.

Determining outcomes

The process of determining outcomes moves beyond the domain of the theory to explore how the theory applied in practice affects the practice of the nursing. Some of the most general outcomes are those that are reflected in nursing standards of quality of care. The components of process, structure, and outcomes that are defined to represent "quality" become the variables that are assessed in deliberative application of theory.

Practice goals are sometimes implied or are made explicit as part of the theory. For example, if the relationships of the theory are claimed to evolve from a sense of community among the elderly or if this seems like a reasonable inference, this general practice goal can become the outcome that is assessed in order to estimate how "well" the theory works to achieve this goal.

Implementing a formal method of study

The methods that are used for this process draw on traditional research methods but shift to include the methods of evaluation and action-oriented research. In this type of research, the method is designed to provide evidence of the effect of the new approach on the overall well-being of people who receive care, on the technical and professional aspects of the practice of nursing, and on the practice setting. Therefore the setting itself becomes a major focus for observation.

If, for example, you have a theory of pain alleviation that you wish to apply in practice, you might design a study that would first estimate the quality of nursing care that is provided before the theory is applied in practice. Your assessment could include the perspective of nurses, people receiving nursing care, and the administrators of the agency. After you have this information, you would begin to use the theory in practice and over time continue to observe the same indicators of quality of care. On the basis of your findings, you could make recommendations for practice, and well as for revisions in the conceptualizations of the theory.

CONCLUSION

The interrelated processes for theory development include creating conceptual meaning, structuring and contextualizing theory, generating and testing theoretic relationships, and deliberative application of theory. Although theory, as we have defined it, can be developed using only conceptual approaches, useful practice theory that assumes research will be generated and theoretic relationships tested. Deliberative application will also occur in practice. It is often useful to describe theory that has already been developed. In Chapter 6 we focus on questions that guide the description of theory.

REFERENCES

Berthold JS: Theoretical and empirical clarification of concepts, Nurs Sci 2(5):406-422, 1964.

Dubin R: Theory building (revised ed), New York, 1978, The Free Press.

Glaser B and Strauss A: The discovery of grounded theory, Chicago, 1967, Aldine Publishing Co.

Newman M: Theory development in nursing, Philadelphia, 1979, FA Davis Co.

Norris CM: Concept clarification in nursing, Rockville, Md, 1982, Aspen Systems Corp.

Reynolds PD: A primer in theory construction, Indianapolis, 1971, The Bobbs-Merrill Company, Inc.

Rogers ME; An introduction to the theoretical basis of nursing, Philadelphia, 1970, FA Davis Co.

Walker LO and Avant KC: Strategies for theory construction in nursing, Norwalk, Conn, 1988, Appleton & Lange.

Wilson J: Thinking with concepts, London, 1963, Cambridge University Press.

6
Description of nursing theory

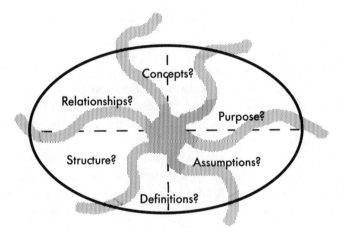

Theory is charactered by certain components that can be
identified, described and organized by asking: What is this? As
this question is posed, understanding begins to form.
Understanding what a theory "is" is essential information for
knowing how a theory works or functions.

The definition of theory we use in this text means that theory is characterized by certain components (see Fig. 4-2). Theoretic components can be identified, described, and organized by asking the critical question: What is this? As this question is posed, understanding of the theory begins to form. Understanding what a theory *is* is essential for critical reflection about how a theory works or functions. This chapter suggests an approach to describing theory. Processes for critical reflection are the focus of Chapter 7.

COMPONENTS OF THEORY

The definition of theory we use implies six descriptive elements. The definition is:

theory A creative and rigorous structuring of ideas that projects a tentative, purposeful, and systematic view of phenomena.

The descriptive components that this definition suggests are:
- *Purpose.* Theory is developed for some reason that can be identified. The purpose of a theory may not be stated explicitly, but one should be identifiable.
- *Concepts.* Theories are structured from ideas expressed as concepts.
- *Definitions.* The concepts of a theory carry identifiable meanings that are conveyed in definitions. Definitions vary in precision and completeness, but conceptual meaning should be identifiable in a theory. The meanings for the concepts created by the theorist give the theory its particular character.
- *Relationships.* Concepts are structured into a systematic form that links each concept with others.
- *Structure.* The relationships between concepts form a whole whereby the ideas of the theory interconnect. The structure makes it possible to follow the reasoning of the theory in its entirety.
- *Assumptions.* Assumptions are the underlying "truths" that determine the nature of concepts, definitions, purpose, relationships, and structure. Many assumptions are difficult to identify because they are implied rather than explicit. Because they are fundamental, we include assumptions as a describable component of theory, even when they are not stated explicitly.

Describing theory is a process of posing questions about these components and responding to the questions with your own "reading" or interpretation of the theory. Some elements will seem clear; others will depend on tentative interpretations. The process of responding to the descriptive questions for each component make it possible to discern that this *is* a theory and what type of theory it is.

POSING QUESTIONS
What is the purpose of this theory?

The general purpose of the theory is important because it specifies the context and situations in which the theory applies. Purpose can be initially approached by asking: "Why is this theory formulated?" Information about the theorist's socio-political context provides insight about circumstances that influenced the creation of the theory. The theorist's experience, the setting in which the theory was formulated, societal trends, philosophic ideas that gave form to the theorist's view, and experience that motivated the creation of the ideas of the theory can all provide insight as to why it was formulated. The responses to this question provide information that pertains to theoretic purposes.

When approaching the question of purpose, it is important to clarify which purposes are embedded in the theoretic structure and which are reasonable extensions of the theory. For example, consider a theory of mother-infant attachment that includes the concepts: (1) ease of delivery, (2) maternal support systems, (3) degree of attachment, and (4) "healthy" infant development. Healthy infant development is an example of a clinical outcome, or purpose, that is embedded in the structure of the theory. The purpose "normal adjustment in later life" represents an extension of the theory, since this concept is not found within the structure of the theory. Purposes that are identifiable within the structure of the theory are usually explicit. Purposes that are reasonable extensions of the theory are important to clarifying the clinical usefulness of the theory, but they are not clearly linked to the central structure of the theory. Purposes outside the context of the theory also suggest directions for further development of the theory.

Some purposes require the practice of nursing in order to be achieved. In these theories the concepts of the theory include nursing actions and behaviors that contribute to the purpose. Pain alleviation and restored self-care ability are examples of purpose that require the practice of nursing and suggest that nursing actions are part of the theory. Note that these purpose statements have a value orientation: "alleviation" and "restoration." These ideas imply change toward a certain goal, not just change for the sake of change. Value connotations such as these are important to understanding the purpose of the theory.

Some purposes may not require the practice of nursing but are useful for understanding phenomena that occur in the context of nursing practice. These purposes can contribute to achieving practice purposes, or they may not be directly relevant to practice goals. Consider, for example, a theory with a central purpose of explaining variables affecting blood flow velocity in the skin. Clinical practice is not necessary to explain blood flow velocity, but a theory with this purpose might be linked to a theoretic explanation of how blood flow velocity influences the incidence of decubiti or the extent of peripheral neuropathy in people with diabetes. A theory that explains skin blood flow velocity would also help practitioners present decubiti and peripheral neuropathy.

Theoretic purposes that do not depend on nursing actions but are of concern to nursing may also involve professional issues in nursing. For example, the purpose of a theory might be to describe features of organizations that empower nurses. This valued and necessary purpose is not directly related to the practice of nursing, but it is certainly useful for changing practice.

Purposes within a theory may be found for individuals or for groups of people. For example, if a theory is developed toward the clinical goal of "pain alleviation," the theory can be examined for purposes appropriate for the nurse, physicians, and family. Consider theory developed with a clinical purpose of "promoting high-level wellness." The role and outcomes for the nurse might be distinctly different from that implied for the person receiving nursing care. The nurse's purpose might be to design a system for recovery. The purpose for the person receiving care might be to recover. Taken together, these two purposes might be viewed as creating an interacting wellness process.

One question that often arises is: "How are purposes to be separated from the concepts of the theory?" Purposes that are part of the matrix of the theory are also concepts of the theory. One approach to identifying which concept is also the central purpose is to describe or to designate the concept toward which theoretic reasoning flows. Ask: "What is the end point of this theory?" and "When is this theory no longer applicable?" Responses to these questions provide clues to purpose and help to clarify the context in which the theory can be used. In Hall's theory (1966), for example, the theory would cease to be valuable when the client was "self-actualized," and self-actualization may be deemed the overall purpose. This purpose of self-actualization represents the end point of theoretic reasoning. In the context of Hall's theory, self-actualization is a purpose that requires nursing actions. Outside the context of Hall's theory, self-actualization is a purpose that is shared with other professions. Hall's theory provides a nursing context within which self-actualization becomes meaningful.

Another question about purpose concerns the individual, family, group, and societal dimensions of the theory. Does the purpose of a theory apply to society? To groups? To individuals? An "adapted society" and an "expanded collective consciousness" are examples of broad purposes that apply to relatively unbounded groups of people. It may be difficult to justify this type of broad scope with respect to nursing purposes. Purposes such as environmental health that apply to communities are broad but clearly within the scope of nursing practice.

What are the concepts of this theory?

Concepts are identified by searching out words or groups of words that represent objects, properties, or events within the theory. You can begin to describe concepts by listing key ideas and tentatively identifying how they seem to relate to one another. As you begin to discern relationships, your perception of the key concepts of the theory will become clearer. One initial difficulty in identifying concepts is identifying which concepts are integral to the theory and which are part of some supporting narrative. There is no easy way to deal with this. By beginning to identify concepts and deriving interrelationships, decisions can be made about which concepts are central to the theory.

As important theoretic concepts are identified, ask questions about the nature of the concepts and their organization. These questions include: "Is there a major concept with subconcepts organized under it?" "Are there several major concepts with subconcepts organized under them?" "Are concepts singular entities?" Are some concepts singular entities and others organized with subconcepts?" "What are the relationships and interrelationships between and among concepts?" "Are some concepts mentioned that do not seem to fit the emerging structure?" Once concepts are identified and questions such as these are addressed, the relationships and structure will begin to emerge.

Questions dealing with the numbers of concepts include: "How many concepts are there?" "How many might be termed 'major' concepts?" "How many are 'minor' concepts?" As you consider the organization and quantity of concepts, address qualitative features of the concepts as well. Questions of quality include: "Do the concepts represent abstractions of objects, properties, or events?" "Is it possible to identify what they represent?" "Are the concepts more empirically grounded, or are they more abstract?" "What proportion of the concepts is empirically grounded?" "What proportion is highly abstract?" "Are the concepts fairly discrete in meaning, or do several have similar meanings?" When similar meanings for concepts exist, ask: "Do they all seem to express a single idea, or are they different?" "How?" Concepts that are alike may represent one central idea that is fairly clear or several different images. For example, the concepts of rehabilitation, restoration, and recovery, which share common meanings, may appear in the same theory with similar meanings or with different meanings.

When you are addressing the question of a theory's concepts, the concepts within it must be examined carefully for quantity, character, emerging relationships, and structure. The description of concepts is crucial because their quantity and character form understanding of the purpose of the theory, the structure and nature of theoretic relationships, the definitions, and the assumptions.

How are the concepts defined?

A "definition" is any explicit or implicit meaning that is conveyed for a concept. Definitions exist to clarify the nature of the abstraction that the theorist constructs in a way that can be comprehended by others. Definitions suggest how word representations of an idea (concept) are expressed in empiric reality.

It is often difficult to determine from a listing of key words which concepts are basic to the theoretic structure and which comprise definitions and assumptions. Carefully reading the theory should provide this information.

Concepts may be defined explicitly (a list of definitions) or implicitly (as part of the narrative, but not labeled as a "definition"). Implied definitions also appear through the context of usage. It is not always easy to recognize implicit definitions, for they are not neatly labeled.

Since concepts may be defined both explicitly and implicitly, ask the following: "How are concepts defined?" "Explicitly?" "Implicitly?" "Both?" "Are implied definitions consistent with explicit definitions?" "Are there key terms with meaning that are defined neither explicitly or implicitly but can be inferred?" "Can common language meanings be taken as the meaning intended?" "Would this approach lead to differing interpretations of the meanings of the concepts?"

Another way to describe definitions is to characterize the extent to which the definitions are general or specific. It is possible for both explicit, implicit, and inferred meanings to be either general or specific. In assessing how general or specific definitions are, ask: "How clearly does the definition suggest an associated empiric experience?" "Is the definition specific about what a phenomena is, or does it suggest what it is used for?" "Does it provide possibilities for empiric indicators that represent the phenomenon?"

For abstract concepts found in many nursing theories, specific definitions are difficult to formulate. Attempting to create specific meanings of "abstract" concepts prematurely may be counterproductive, and definitions that specify general features can conjure up very specific mental images of the actual experience. An early definition that is broad and nonspecific encourages the exploration of many possible meanings. General meanings are also preferred in broad scope theory or theory that is not likely to be empirically "tested." Most definitions have both specific and general features. Ask: "How are definitions both specific and general?"

Once definitions are identified, ask: "Are similar definitions used for different concepts?" "Are differing definitions used for the same concept?" "Are some concepts defined differently from common convention?" " Are definitions expanded as the narrative proceeds?" "Is it difficult to judge whether definitions are provided at all?" "Can definitions fit other terms within or outside of the structure of the theory?"

What is the nature of relationships?

Relationship statements provide links among and between concepts. The nature of relationships in theory may take several forms. Often relationship statements that are uncovered may be peripheral to the core of the theory.

As concepts are identified, ideas about relationships between them begin to form. Suppose you uncover a relationship statement, "The individual is comprised of three dimensions and is an integral part of the environment." This suggests that the individual is related to an environment and that there are three interrelated subcomponents of the individual.

Once a tentative identification of relationships is made, ask: "Are there concepts that stand alone, unrelated to others?" "Are there concepts interrelated with other concepts in several ways and others related in only one or two ways?" "Are there concepts to which several other concepts relate but that, in turn, are not related to other concepts?"

The ways in which the relationships emerge provide clues to the theoretic purposes and the assumptions on which the theory is based. Some concepts may be linked to the theory by assumptions. This may explain why the concept seems to fit within the matrix of the theory, but a theoretic relationship containing the concept is not explicitly stated. The theoretic purpose can be represented by the one-way relationships of several concepts with one specific concept that in turn is not linked to any other concepts (that is, the links end with this specific concept). As links between concepts are identified, you can address the nature or character of relationships. If a relationship is unclear, you should include inferences about the possible relationships and their character; your ideas can provide clues for further development of the theory.

Examine the nature of relationships by asking: "Are the relationships basically descriptive, or do they explain?" "Do they create meaning without explaining?" "Do they impart understanding?" "Is there evidence that some relationships are predictive?" Relationships within theory that create meaning and impart understanding often link multiple concepts in a loose structure. In other forms of description, concepts are interrelated without elaboration on how and why conceptual relationships are arranged. Concepts that are interrelated to explain often convey how empiric events occur and may provide some detail about how and why concepts interrelate. Prediction implies if-then statements about the occurrence of empiric phenomena. When predictions are shown to be valid, they are usually based on explanation.

The statement, "Individuals are comprised of three dimensions," is mainly descriptive. It implies that one concept, the individual, is comprised of three parts called dimensions. If expanded to "The individual is comprised of three dimensions that overlap and share common core areas," the statement becomes more explanatory. It proposes that each dimension had a shared area with another dimension and that there is an area shared by all three. When "interrelated whole" is added, the "how" of the relationship becomes even clearer, for the dimensions must overlap to interrelate the parts of the individual. Predictions are fairly easy to detect. Sentences that translate into "if-then" statements are predictive. It is not possible to make an "if-then" statement out of "The individual is comprised of three dimensions" unless it is the implied, "If not three dimensions, then not the individual." The statement, "The individual is an interrelated whole comprised of three dimensions that overlap and share common areas," implies that disturbances in one sphere would be reflected in other spheres. This prediction, however, is not explicit.

Suppose the statement read: "Because the individual is an interrelated whole comprised of three dimensions that overlap and share common areas, a disturbance in one dimension is reflected in disturbances in other dimensions." This statement is clearly predictive. The distinctions between description, explanation, and prediction are not always clear. Generally description means that the statement projects *what* something is or features of its character. Explanation suggests *how* or *why* it is. Prediction projects circumstances that create or alter a phenomenon. Our use of "descriptive," "explanatory," and "predictive" in describing the nature of theoretic relationships refers only to the form of the theory. In this context, we do not mean to imply that empiric validation or "findings" are required to discern whether relationship statements are descriptive, explanatory, or predictive.

What is the structure of the theory?

The structure of theory gives overall form to the conceptual relationships within it. The structure emerges from the relationships of the theory. Consider two concepts within a theory: "individual" and "environment." In one theory individuals are part of the environment, and in another individuals are separate from the environment. In both theories there is an identifiable relationship between individuals and environment; however, the structure of the relationship differs, as symbolically represented in Fig. 6-1. Since a relationship between two theoretic concepts can take different structural forms, it is important to describe the nature of both.

Although your responses to questions concerning the relationships of theory usually suggest the form, in some cases they do not. Many theories do not contain a single discernible structure where all concepts fit into a coherent, unified network. There may be several, perhaps competing, structures that cannot be reconciled. Determining the structure of theory will be difficult if the network of relationships is unclear or very complex. Fig. 6-2 depicts a sample of four structural forms and the ideas they suggest. Some theories may reflect one or more of these structures, whereas others will not. Sometimes individual concepts within theories may be structured in these forms. Structural forms are powerful devices for shaping our perceptions of reality.

Consider how you might structure the relationship statement, "Individuals are comprised of component parts." This only suggests a structure in which parts are perceptible, and any image on Fig. 6-2 could represent it

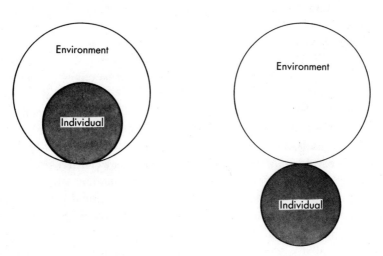

FIG. 6-1
Alternate structure forms for individual-environment relationships.

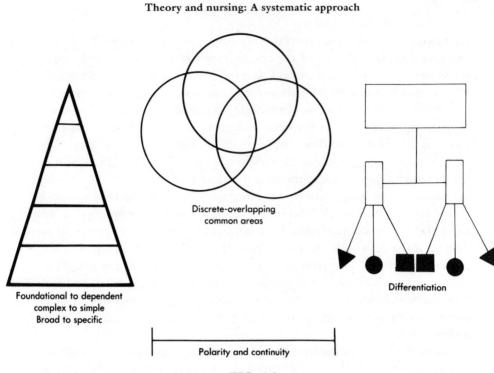

Foundational to dependent
complex to simple
Broad to specific

Discrete-overlapping
common areas

Differentiation

Polarity and continuity

FIG. 6-2
Structural idea forms.

except the one that suggests polarity. Suppose each of these structures represents the broad theory of "health." The triangular drawing suggests that health is comprised of a series of related subconcepts that vary in breadth or simplicity. It also suggests foundational concepts on which other subconcepts are built. The base level might be genetic integrity, followed by organ-system health, and finally health of communities or societies. A theory that deals with how genetic "health" forms the basis for individual, collective, and societal "health" might be structured in the preceding manner.

The overlapping circles depict discrete components that have common areas between and among them. "Health" might be viewed as having biophysiologic, psychoemotional, and sociocultural aspects. If a person is biologically well but psychoemotionally unwell, the diagram suggests that illness will affect biophysiologic wellness. Psychoemotional ill health could result in biophysiologic consequences. Basically the overlapping circles illustrate that, although health is comprised of separate components, there is sharing between any two components, as well as among all three. The structure as illustrated suggests an equality in importance, overlap, and sharing among the three subunits.

Development of nursing theory

Applying this idea to the horizontal line drawing on the figure shows "health" represented as a continuum. This structure suggests that health is in a linear relationship with illness. When health is placed on a continuum with illness on the opposite end, health is conceptualized as a continuous variable, and degrees of health and illness are possible. The extremes of a continuum also suggest that health is the absence of illness and illness is the absence of health. If health is viewed as a concept that is continuous with illness, health and illness can be represented by a continuum. If health and illness are considered as entirely different concepts, they do not fit this structural form. A relationship between gender and society could not be represented on a continuum, for example.

The fourth structural form conveys the idea of differentiation, dividing major concepts into subconcepts. For this structural form, health might be differentiated into its mental and physical aspects. Physical health could be further divided into "anatomic" health and "physiologic" health, with some comparable division such as "emotion" and "spirit" for mental health. Differentiation can proceed indefinitely. Some concepts lend themselves to differentiation more easily than others. "Needs" is a concept that can be easily differentiated, whereas the concept of "holism" cannot.

As you study the examples of structure, note how different concepts fit some structures more easily than others and how some concepts such as "holistic health" cannot be represented by any of them. Structures for representing health may not make sense for you because they are not consistent with your personal ideas about its nature.

As relationships are explored, the overall theoretic structure and the structure of individual components begin to emerge. To address questions of structure, begin by asking: "What are the most central relationships?" "What is the direction, strength, and quality of relationships?" "Can I draw a model that shows the structure of the theory?" "What is the order of appearance of relationships within the narrative?" "Do relationships appear to move toward or away from the theoretic purpose?" "Do relationships coalesce concepts or differentiate them?" "Does the theorist diagram the structure?"

Once the structure of the major or central relationships is identified, other aspects of structure can be described. Ask: "How are other structures united with central or core relationships?" "Can all relationships be structured?" "Do the structures take multiple forms?" "Are competing or partial structures suggested?" "Does the theorist provide diagrams that illustrate aspects of structure?"

Once you have structured the relationships, describe the entire structural form. Notice how the relationships move as the theory unfolds. A theory that defies structuring can sometimes be approached by simply outlining the order in which concepts are presented. Outlining can provide insight about how ideas are organized. Some recognizable structure is essential to theory, for structure flows from relationships.

On what assumptions does the theory build?

Assumptions are those basic givens or accepted "truths" that are fundamental to theoretic reasoning. In order to uncover assumptions, a central question is: "What is the author taking as truth or as an accepted value?" This question can be asked once the purposes are determined, the concepts are structured by relational statements, and the definitions described.

Sometimes the theorist states assumptions explicitly. If so, ask: "What are they?" "What do they assume?" Statements explicitly labeled "assumptions" may not be the same as the assumptions that are basic to the theory. The extent to which explicitly labeled assumptions *are* assumptions and not something else must be examined. It is often difficult to separate assumptions that are implicit or integrated into the narrative of the theory from relationship statements, but they must be identified. As with explicit assumptions, ask: "What are they?" "What do they assume?"

To further explore your ideas about the assumptions of the theory, ask: "What individual, environment, nursing, and health-related assumptions are made?" "Are assumptions competing or compatible?" "Are there several assumptions about one phenomena and few about another?" "Are assumptions made at the outset, between and within relationships, or in relation to the purposes of the theory?"

Assumptions may take the form of factual assertions, or they may reflect value positions. Factual assumptions are those knowable or potentially knowable by empiric experience. Value assumptions assert or imply what is right, good, or ought to be. Often an empirically knowable assumption such as, "It is assumed for the purposes of this theory that people want information," contains important underlying value assumptions. The assumption that people want information (which could be empirically verified) may further imply that "information is good to have," which cannot be verified empirically. It is important to examine factual assumptions by asking: "What value does this factual assumption reflect?" It is also important to examine all other components of theory and ask: "What does this concept, definition, relationship, structure, or purpose assume?"

Once you discern assumptions, the values held by the theorist can be explored by asking: "What does the theorist assume to be valuable, good, right, wrong, or worthwhile?" "Are there value-laden terms and phrases in the definitions of concepts and in the supporting narrative of the theory?"

"Who is assumed to be responsible for the experiences or circumstances of the theoretic reality?" "Who benefits from the circumstances or experiences of this theory?" These questions often give clues to values that form fundamental assumptions. For example, the Freudian theoretic notion of "penis envy" implies that penises are body parts that are so valued as to be enviable. It further implies that people who do not have a penis will experience this value-laden emotion. A useful approach to uncovering hidden values is to imagine possibilities other than that presented in the theory. If these alternate possibilities are quite plausible, and not simply ridiculous, you have uncovered important value assumptions. Imagining the idea of "womb envy," which is not a part of Freudian thinking, but is a plausible alternate possibility, indicates that you have uncovered an important androcentric assumption from which the theory builds.

The descriptive component of assumptions is often based on ideas taken so much for granted that they are difficult to recognize. An example of such an obvious assumption is that "reality is what can be perceived and experienced through the senses." This assumption is fundamental to empirics, but it is not an assumption of other patterns of knowing.

Sometimes it is not possible to accept a theory because it is unusual or unfamiliar. Uneasiness or discomfort with a theory is sometimes a clue to assumptions that are unlike your own beliefs or values. Once assumptions are recognized, the theory containing them can be understood on its own terms.

Forming a complete description

In summary, the five questions for describing theory are:
- What is the purpose of this theory? This question addresses why the theory was formulated and reflects the contexts and situations to which the theory can be applied.
- What are the concepts of this theory? This question identifies the ideas that are structured and related within the theory. It questions the qualitative and quantitative dimensions of concepts.
- How are the concepts defined? This question clarifies the meaning for concepts within the theory. It questions how empiric experience is represented by the ideas within the theory.
- What is the nature of relationships? This question addresses how concepts are linked together. It focuses on the various forms relationship statements can take and how they give form to the theory.
- What is the structure of the theory? This question addresses the overall form of the conceptual interrelationships. It discerns whether the theory contains partial structures or has one basic form.

- On what assumptions does the theory build? This question addresses the basic truths that underlie theoretic reasoning. It questions whether assumptions reflect philosophic values or factual assertions.

A general approach that can be used in describing theory is to read the work and then begin to consider the descriptive questions. The outline shown in the box on pp. 121 and 122 summarizes the questions that can be asked to form a complete description of theory. All questions are not necessarily answerable for a single theory. As you respond to the questions, concepts will be tentatively identified, and the purpose of the theory will emerge. The definitions will become evident, and you will begin to see relationships. From the nature of the relationships, you will be able to address questions concerning the structure of the theory. Responses to questions concerning assumptions provide a level of awareness of meanings and will help you form understanding of the theory. After an initial description of components, each component is reexamined and revised. There is no best way to approach the task, and each nurse develops a scheme that suits individual style.

For any theory, it is not easy to describe the theoretic purpose and assumptions, and the description is usually tentative, but these components can be found. Concepts and their definitions are more readily identifiable, especially those that are explicit. Often discerning relationships and structure is a problematic area in describing theory, but these traits will be present in the work if it is a theory.

Forming a complete description of theory requires systematic and critical examination of the work. Often every word, phrase, and sentence must be examined for meaning. Ideas that emerge in response to the descriptive questions often lead to uncertainty and revisions of earlier ideas. After a time the description does begin to take shape, and fewer changes occur. There will always be some tentativeness in your descriptions because your description requires your own interpretive insights with respect to the theorist's ideas and these insights change. If you are not able to reach a tentative resolution with respect to the fundamental nature of a theory after reasonable study and thought, the best course of action is to propose your ideas for revision and further development of the theory. Your continuing uncertainty indicates that further theoretic development must occur.

ADDITIONAL ELEMENT OF DESCRIPTION: SCOPE

For some purposes it may be important to describe the breadth or the scope of the theory. Scope is not a structural component of theory per se, but it can be considered a structural trait. It is sometimes important to describe

GUIDE FOR THE DESCRIPTION OF THEORY

1. Purpose
- Why is this theory formulated?
- Is there an overall purpose for the theory? A hierarchy of purposes? Separate numerous purposes?
- Is there a purpose for the nurse? Society? Environment?
- How broad or narrow is the purpose?
- What is the value orientation of the purpose? Positive, negative, neutral?
- Does achieving the theoretic purpose require a nursing context?
- Does/do the purpose/purposes reflect understanding? Creation of meaning? Description, explanation, and prediction of phenomena?
- When would the theory cease to be applicable? What is the "end point?"
- What purpose not explicitly embedded in the matrix of the theory can be identified?

2. Concepts
- Is there one major concept with subconcepts organized under it?
- How many concepts are there?
- How many major ones?
- How many minor ones?
- Can the concepts be ordered, related? Arranged into any configuration? Are there concepts that cannot be interrelated?
- Are concepts broad in scope? Narrow?
- How abstract or empiric are the concepts?
- What is the balance between highly abstract and highly empiric concepts?
- Do concepts represent objects, properties, events? Can you say? Are there concepts that are closely related?

3. Definitions
- Which concepts are defined? Which are not?
- Are concepts defined explicitly? Implicitly?
- Can definitions be inferred from contextual usage?
- Which concepts are defined specifically? Generally?
- Are there competing definitions for some concepts? Are there similar definitions for different concepts?
- Do any explicit defined concepts not need definition?
- Are any concepts defined contrary to common convention?

Continued.

GUIDE FOR THE DESCRIPTION OF THEORY—cont'd.

4. Relationships

- What are the major relationships within the theory?
- Which relationships are obvious? Which are implied?
- Do relationships include all concepts? Which are not included?
- Are some concepts included in multiple relationships?
- Is there a hierarchy of relationships? Do relationships create meaning and understanding? Do they do this by describing, explaining? Predicting? What mix of each?
- Are relationships directional? What is their direction? Are they neutral?
- Are there mixed, competing, or incongruous relationships?
- Are relationships illustrated?

5. Structure

- How are overall and individual ideas organized?
- If outlined, what would the theory look like?
- Do relationships expand concepts into larger wholes or vice versa? Do they link concepts in a linear fashion?
- Does the structure move concepts away from or toward the purposes?
- Are there several structures that emerge? What is their form? Do they fit together?
- Could more than one structure represent the overall structural relationships?
- Where is there no structure?

6. Assumptions

- What assumptions underlie the theory? Are assumptions explicit, implicit, or derivable from context and meanings?
- What are the individual, nurse, society, environment, and health assumed to be like?
- Do assumptions have an obvious value orientation? What is it?
- Could assumptions be factually verified?
- Where are assumptions located within the structure? Prior to, within, or following theoretic reasoning?
- Can assumptions be hierarchically arranged or otherwise ordered?
- Do assumptions have any identifiable relationship to theoretic relationships or structure?
- Are there competing assumptions?

the scope of theory because its scope reflects its usefulness for practice and research purposes. Also, traditional typologies for describing theory such as *micro* and *macro* require knowing the scope of the theory. The purposes and concepts are key elements when the scope of theory is described.

The scope of a theory refers to the breadth or range of phenomena to which the theory applies. The level of abstraction of the concepts of the theory is integral to its scope. Theory may be characterized as *micro, macro, molecular, midrange, molar, atomistic,* and *holistic. Grand theory* is a term also found in the literature, meaning theory that covers broad areas of concern within a discipline. *Meta theory* is a term used to designate theory about theory and the processes for developing theory.

Categorizations of scope are relative, and labels that are typically used to classify the scope of theory reflect a continuum of breadth. "Micro," "molecular," and "atomistic", for example, suggest relatively narrow-range phenomena, whereas "macro" and "molar" imply that the theory covers a relatively broader range of phenomena. These categories are often relative to the scope of the discipline. What is micro for one discipline may be midrange in others. A theory of holistic humans would likely be broad in scope in almost any discipline and would deal with patterns reflecting the whole. Grand theory, unlike macro and molar theory, refers to very broad-scope theory in most disciplines. The term "atomistic" implies a narrow scope and has the connotation of assuming that parts are a legitimate focus for study in order to generalize about the whole. Conversely, "holistic" connotes that the sum of parts cannot reflect the whole.

Fig. 6-3 depicts these theory classifications relative to each other on a breadth continuum. There are no predetermined criteria for determining whether a theory is micro or macro, molecular, midrange or molar. At best these words are guides.

Two descriptive components of theory can be used as a basis for determining where a theory is placed in terms of breadth: purpose and concepts. For theoretic purposes ask, "How broad are they?" The following illustrate a narrowing scope of purpose:

- Expansion of consciousness
- High-level wellness
- Recovery from illness
- Pain alleviation
- Improving regional blood flow
- Increasing amplitude and frequency of action potential on nerve fiber bundles

Micro or molecular theory may reflect purposes that can only be known indirectly because evidence to validate their achievement requires percep-

Theory and nursing: A systematic approach

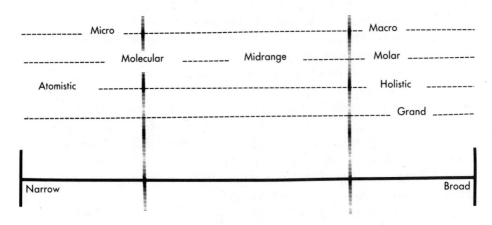

FIG. 6-3

**Relative classification of theory based on breadth of concepts
and goal statements.**

tions keener than those provided by unaided senses. The purpose of altering action potential is representative of this category. Improving regional blood flow is an even broader purpose than altering action potential, since in some cases it is indirectly perceptible, whereas action potentials cannot be assessed without sensitive signal processing equipment. Concepts contained in such theories are narrow and often specifically defined.

When the purpose increases in scope to represent a portion of an accepted overall purpose for a profession or discipline, midrange theory is being approached. Theory of pain alleviation is an example of this range, for pain alleviation is one of several areas of concern to nursing. Micro theories might attempt to explain the physiology of pain phenomena, whereas midrange theories would deal with pain alleviation as a segment of nursing's total interest. Concepts contained in midrange theory reflect this "part of whole" orientation; they are broader than those contained in micro theories but still do not reflect the totality of nursing's concern.

Macro theories conceptualize purpose broadly. Health, expanded consciousness, and high-level wellness, not just for individuals but for people in general, are examples of such purposes. Macro theories deal with the whole of nursing's concern. Concepts within these theories tend to be broad in scope and related to individuals as wholes rather than as portions of the person's structure or function.

An example may serve to illustrate how purpose and concepts interrelate to provide information that can be used in responding to questions about scope. Abdellah et al. (1960) have proposed that nursing purposes can be described as the solution of problems in 21 different categories (Abdellah et al. 1960). Each problem is complex in itself, and taken together they are represented as the totality of nursing function. Problem 11 is: "to facilitate maintenance of sensory function." Theory regarding the solution and prevention of this problem could be considered midrange theory, since it is only one of 21 others of concern to nursing. Narrower theory is possible concerning the development or maintenance of sensory function in diverse groups such as those with chronic illness, the young or aged, or any of numerous subdivisions. Theory of sensory neural transport would represent micro theory in relation to this problem area. Assume that the maintenance of function in all 21 problem areas constitutes health, whereas the solution of existing problems constitutes movement from illness toward health, with health being a valued purpose for individuals. Macro theory would be theory that interrelates all 21 problem areas so that the general purpose of health restoration or maintenance could be approached.

There are diverse points of view concerning the appropriate scope for theories in nursing. Regardless of the breadth that is desired or sought, the purpose should help achieve an accepted nursing purpose. If the goal is to alleviate pain, theory and research that focuses on nerve action potentials can be justified with respect to its link to the nursing practice goal of alleviating pain.

Broad purposes may be achieved by linking narrower theories or by initially formulating broad theory. The assumptions and values orientation underlying both approaches differ. Many persons believe that a reductionistic approach (linking parts to explain the whole) is not desirable. Others state that molar theories are not useful for directing research or practice and must be "reduced" before laboratory testing and practice application. Given the range and complexity of nursing's purposes, a range of breadth or scope of theories is needed.

CONCLUSION

Theory can be described on the basis of its purpose, concepts, definitions, relationships, structure, and assumptions. Describing theory requires careful study of the work and interpretive responses to questions concerning descriptive elements of the theory. Each of these components is derived from the definition of theory used within this text. Once theory is thoughtfully described, critical questions can be addressed that reveal ideas concerning its function. These questions are considered in Chapter 7.

REFERENCES

Abdellah FG, et al: Patient-centered approaches to nursing, New York, 1960, The MacMillan Co.

Hall LE: Another view of nursing care and quality. In Straub KM and Parker KS, editors: Continuity of patient care: the role of nursing, Washington DC, 1966, Catholic University Press, pp 47-60.

7

Critical reflection of nursing theory

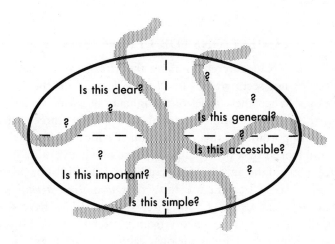

Critical reflection is a process that asks how well a theory serves some purpose. The nature of theory, as revealed with critical reflection, is basic to choosing theory to guide research, practice, and education.

Describing and critically reflecting theory are fundamentally different processes. Description can be compared to setting forth "facts" about theory or asking, "What is this?" Critical reflection, on the other hand, involves ascertaining how well a theory serves some purpose. Critical reflection is a process that asks: How does it (theory) function or work? For what purpose?

In this chapter we identify questions that can be used in critical reflection. As you question how a theory works, you will gain insight about how theory might be used and how it might be further developed to form understanding.

QUESTIONS FOR REFLECTION

As you study and read different nursing theories, you may have thoughts like: "This does not seem right," or "Maybe I could do this" or "This is really exciting." When these types of thoughts occur, what you are doing is comparing the theory to some personal and perhaps unrecognized ideas about what is important for theory. Each nurse's ideas of the adequacy of a theory are influenced by a personal perspective of what is valuable or good. For *research* you might agree: "This could be helpful." For *practice,* you might think: "Maybe I could use this." For *idea stimulation,* you might think: "This is really exciting." In these instances you have formed an impression of the value of the theory from personal values about practice, research, and critical thinking. Your own values are important components that contribute to a more formal critical reflection process.

Critical reflection contributes to developing ideas about how well the theory relates to practice, research, or educational activities. Members of a discipline form ideas about what questions to ask and what responses are generally accepted if a theory is to be seen as valuable for the discipline. Just as there are many ways to describe theory, there are many critical questions that can be asked about the functional value of theory and many responses to these questions. Once the questions are asked, members of a discipline can consider what responses they tend to value and why. The questions we suggest are organized around characteristics of theory. These characteristics form the basis for considering the merits and shortcomings of a theory in relation to some purpose. The questions we pose are consistent with generally accepted methods for evaluating theories that have been described in the nursing literature. (Ellis, 1968; Fawcett, 1989; Hardy, 1974; Stevens, 1990). A theory is examined with respect to each of the questions, and the responses to the questions are used to form conclusions about how well the theory serves some purpose.

The questions for critical reflection are:

- How clear is this theory?
- How simple is this theory?
- How general is this theory?
- How accessible is this theory?
- How important is this theory?

There are no "correct" answers to these questions, and the questions do not imply the responses. For example, the question "How clear is this?" does not necessarily mean that a theory "should" be perfectly clear. Rather, the people who address the question use it as a tool to focus on issues of clarity and gain understanding of how this might contribute to the theory's function for a particular purpose. As you engage in discussions that are centered around the questions, you can form a consensus with your colleagues as to where to go next in developing the theory. These insights can best be formed in discussion among people with diverse perspectives. For example, even though a theory that challenges assumptions about practice is somewhat unclear, it may be an important theory for changing nursing practice and provide new concepts with which to work. The fact that it is not clear is part of its strength.

Although each of the five critical reflection questions is fundamentally different, you will find that they are interrelated. For example, one question addresses accessibility, and another addresses generality. If a theory is seen as general or broad in scope, it may be less accessible (less related to empiric reality) than if it were narrower in scope (less general).

Responses to the description questions in Chapter 6 affect your responses to the critical reflection questions. For example, to decide how clear, accessible, or general a theory is, you need to describe some purpose of the theory, what concepts are included, and how they are structured. As your description of theory is formed, you can begin the process of critical reflection. The ideas you develop from this process contribute to your own critical insights, as well as to substantive discussion that forms directions for theory development.

How clear is this theory?

In addressing this question, you will be considering semantic clarity, semantic consistency, structural clarity, and structural consistency. Clarity, in general, refers to how well the theory can be understood and how consistently the ideas are conceptualized. Semantic clarity and consistency primarily refer to the understandability of theoretic meaning as it relates to concepts. Structural clarity and consistency reflects the understandability of connections between concepts within the theory.

Semantic clarity. The definitions of concepts in the theory are an important aspect of semantic clarity. Definitions help to establish empiric meaning for concepts within the theory. If concepts are not defined or are incompletely defined, the empiric indicators for the idea become less clear. When concepts are clearly defined, identification of empiric indicators is relatively easy. Clarity implies, in part, that, when different nurses read the theory, a similar empiric reality comes to mind when the word for the concept is used. If there are no definitions or if only a few of the concepts are defined, clarity will be limited.

Types of definitions that are used within theory affect semantic clarity. When definitions reflect both specific and general traits, clarity is enhanced, whereas a general or a specific definition alone often limits clarity. Specific definitions lend clarity because they provide clear and accurate guidance for the intended empiric indicators for a concept. General definitions contribute a contextual sense of meaning for concepts, lending a richness of meaning that is not possible when concepts are specifically defined. Considering the extent to which each type of definition contributes to clarity of meaning can help you form your own ideas about the adequacy of the theory for your purpose.

Clarity may be obscured by borrowing terms from other disciplines or by using common language terms that carry broad general meanings. Words such as "stress" or "coping" have general common language meanings, and they also have specific theoretic meanings in other disciplines. If words with multiple meanings are used in theory and not defined, a person's everyday meaning of the term is taken to be what is meant in the theory. If people consistently understand a term to be one thing and the theorist intends another meaning, clarity is lost. Clarity is enhanced when the concept is defined consistently with common meanings of the term within the profession.

Clarity is affected when words are used that have no common meaning or when words are invented or coined by the theorist to represent some idea. Coined words can help to convey a meaning for which there is no word. Coined or new words can detract from clarity, especially when a more familiar word or phrase would suffice. It would be possible to generate an entire theory about "quizzendroids," "plankerods," and "ziots." The theory could be "logical" and consistent but unclear because the words are invented and have no meaning. Although this is an exaggerated example, it demonstrates the effects on clarity when vague or strange words are used, when words are not defined, or when words are used with many possible meanings.

Semantic clarity can also be affected by excessive verbiage. Normally, varying words to represent similar meanings is a writing skill that can be used to avoid overuse of a single term. But in theory, if several similar concepts are used interchangeably when one would suffice, there is excess verbiage. When words with similar meaning are used to represent the central concepts of a theory, the clarity of the presentation of the theory is reduced rather than improved. In theory, varying the word for important concepts interjects subtly different meanings. For example, interchanging the words "restoration," "rehabilitation," and "recovery" for the same concept changes clarity, since each word has a slightly different meaning.

Clarity is also affected when excessive narrative is included. Semantic clarity may be decreased by use of excessive examples; however, the judicious use of examples usually aids clarity. Diagrams can enhance or obscure clarity. To enhance clarity diagrams should be self explanatory and simple in expression, because overly complex illustrations discourage comprehension. In general, the alternate mode of providing information in the form of diagrams will help make the ideas in the theory clearer.

Economy of words, key definitions, and wise use of examples and diagrams lend clarity. Absolute semantic clarity can never be achieved, nor is it necessarily desirable. Because of the limitations of language, no matter how clearly the theorist represents theoretic meaning, it will not be perceived uniformly by all readers.

Semantic consistency. Semantic consistency is a second feature to consider with respect to the question of clarity. A theory that is inconsistently presented leads to confusion. Semantic consistency means that the concepts of the theory are used in ways that are consistent with their definition. Sometimes a definition is explicitly stated, and somewhere within the theory another meaning is implied. When key words are not explicitly defined, their implied meanings may be inconsistent from one usage to the next. Occasionally words are explicitly defined in different ways. Inconsistencies that occur when terms are defined explicitly are fairly easy to uncover, but other types of inconsistencies may be more covert.

The consistent use of basic assumptions is important in achieving consistency. The theory's purpose, definitions of concepts, and relationships need to be consistent with the stated assumptions of the theory. Examples and diagrams can also be considered in light of the assumptions of the theory. Suppose, for example, a basic theoretic assumption is the unity of persons and environment and that both change simultaneously and irreversibly through time and space. This assumption is consistent with a definition of health as expanding consciousness, but inconsistent with a theoretic conceptualization of health as a state of adaptation. Adaptation typically implies conforming or adjusting to environmental stimuli in order to "fit within" the environment. The concept of adaptation tends to suggest the assumption that events external to the person are primary as a determinant of health and that the person and the environment are separate entities. Unity of person and environment is a concept that can be used to convey an assumption that humans and environment are interconnected and change simultaneously. Simultaneous change negates the idea of conforming or adjusting to a stimuli as health, but rather implies incorporating change, becoming a different person, and increasing options and awareness of choice.

The purposes of the theory must be consistent with all other components. A purpose of health, achieved by deliberate nursing actions, may be at odds with the basic assumption that "health is deterministic." The purpose in this example is to create something that is assumed to be deterministic and therefore cannot be influenced by deliberate acts. Becoming aware of this inconsistency helps to clarify other meanings that are conveyed in the definitions and other components of the theory.

In reflecting on consistency, you can examine your descriptions for each component of theory and consider where there are consistencies and inconsistencies within, as well as between, the descriptive elements of the theory. Definitions must be examined for consistency with each other and in relation to assumptions. Structure is sometimes inconsistent with relationships. If a theory is extremely inconsistent, it is difficult to address other reflective questions concerning the theory. Some semantic inconsistencies within theory are more common early in their development and leave room for new possibilities for further development. However, inconsistencies at the basic roots of theory, as between assumptions and goals, have implications that will affect the entire theory and must be addressed.

Structural clarity. Structural clarity is closely linked to semantic clarity. Structural clarity refers to how understandable the connections and reasoning within theory are. The descriptive elements of structure and relationships provide important information for addressing this dimension of clarity.

In a theory with structural clarity, you can readily recognize the underlying conceptual network. With structural clarity, concepts are interconnected and organized into a coherent whole. If you cannot discern the structure of the theory, you begin to search for those structural elements that are related, and where the gaps occur in the flow of the theory. If all major relationships are included within a single structure, clarity is enhanced. Clarity is lost if there are gaps so that the relationships are not contained within a coherent structure. Pieces of relationships, rudiments of structure, or concepts that stand alone are evidence that parts have not yet been integrated into the whole during the development of the theory. When major concepts do not fit within the structure, clarity is significantly obscured.

Structural consistency. Structural consistency relates to the use of different structural forms within theory. Usually theory is built around one predominant structural form. Sometimes one form provides the general profile for the conception of the relationships of theory, and subcomponents of the theory take a somewhat different form. Whatever the structure, consistency throughout the theory with respect to the structure serves as a conceptual "map" that enhances clarity. A theorist may begin with a structural movement that is linear. If this structure is reflected in the relationships as the theory develops, you will observe a high level of structural consistency. A shift in reasoning to a structure of differentiation may be confusing, or the reasoning might function well within the overall structure.

In summary, the question, "How clear is this theory?" can be used to explore in what ways a theory is clear and comprehensible, how it is not, and what its level of clarity means for the development of the theory. The ideas of semantic and structural consistency and clarity can be used to guide discussion of issues of clarity. A very general (broad scope) theory may be quite ambiguous, but useful in stimulating new ideas. A midrange theory of hopelessness, for example, may have aspects that are vague, but still be important in helping nurses understand the experience. However, the ambiguity of that same theory may affect its usefulness for guiding research. Becoming aware of the ways in which clarity is obscured in light of your purpose makes it possible to design ways to further develop its clarity. The degree to which a theory must be clear depends on how the nurse intends to use it.

How simple is this theory?

Complexity implies many theoretic relationships between and among numerous concepts. On the other hand, theoretic simplicity means that the number of elements within each descriptive category, particularly concepts and their interrelationships, are minimal.

The following example illustrates theoretic simplicity. Suppose that a theory contained three major concepts: A, B, and C. A theory interrelating these concepts would be quite simple, since only three interrelationships would be possible: A and B, A and C, and B and C. Adding subconcepts 1 and 2 to each of A, B, and C (e.g., A1, A2) would leave the theorist with three major concepts (A, B, and C) and six subconcepts for a total of nine. A theorist working with nine concepts has greater theoretic complexity than a theorist working with only three concepts. Adding even one or two concepts to a theory greatly increases potential for theoretic interrelationships and, subsequently, complexity.

The desirability of simplicity or complexity varies with the stage of theory development. In grounded theory, for example, there may be considerable complexity as the theory begins to emerge, but, as it develops, relationships and concepts are coalesced, and the theory becomes more simple. Regardless of approach to theory development, some concepts created early in the process may eventually be deleted or changed. In the above example, suppose concepts A, A1, and A2 came to be seen as unimportant in relation to the theory's purpose. The theoretic complexity added by A and its subconcepts could be removed, and only the simpler relationships between B and C and their subconcepts would remain.

Theories reflect varying degrees of simplicity. In nursing, some situations suggest the need for relatively simple and broad theory that can be used as a general guide for practice. Other situations suggest simple but more empirically accessible theory to guide research. Still other situations suggest the need for theory that is relatively complex, because of the value such theory has for enhancing understanding of extremely complex practice situations.

How general is this theory?

The generality of a theory refers to its breadth of scope; a general theory can be applied to a broad array of situations. Generality is reflected by the scope of concepts and purposes within the theory. Parsimony is sometimes used as a synonym to describe the trait of theoretic simplicity, but the concept of parsimony also includes the idea of generality. A parsimonious theory is one that is conceptually simple but accounts for a broad range of empiric experiences.

The scope of concepts and purposes within the theory provide clues to its generality. A theory containing broad concepts will encompass more ideas with fewer words than one containing very narrow concepts. Concepts of "humans" and "universe" could be interpreted as organizing almost every fact or idea possible. A comprehensive theory with these two concepts would be highly generalizable. A theory interrelating a single person and the physical environment is less general, although still fairly broad in scope. The concept "individual" implies that the theory is concerned with a single person. The use of "physical" as a modifier to "environment" conveys the notion of environment in part only. Information about individuals in communities could not be understood within this theory. A theory relating characteristics of acutely ill people with the intensive care unit environment is even less general, and the scope of concepts narrows.

Questions that address the generality of theory include: "To whom does this theory apply, and when does it apply?" "Is the purpose one that pertains to all health care professionals?" "To people in general?" "Does the purpose apply to specific specialties of nursing and only at given times?" The more limited the scope of application of the theory, the less general the theory.

Whether or not generality is viewed as desirable depends on the purpose of the theory. General theory organizes many ideas and is quite useful for generating ideas or hypothesis. Nursing theories that address broad concepts such as individuals, society, health, and environment have a high degree of generality and are useful for organizing ideas about universal health behaviors. Theories that address a specific human experience such as pain are less general and, because of their relative specificity, are useful for guiding practice in a clinical setting.

How accessible is this theory?

Accessibility addresses the extent to which empiric indicators can be identified for concepts within the theory. It also refers to how attainable the projected outcomes of the theory are. If a theory is to be used for explaining and predicting some aspect of the practice world, its theoretic concepts must be linked to empiric indicators. Concepts can be made empirically accessible through generating and testing relationships, deliberative application of theory, and clarifying conceptual meaning.

Only selected dimensions of highly abstract concepts may be empirically accessible. If the concepts of a theory do not reflect empiric dimensions or if the empiric dimensions are very obscure, they may be ideas that cannot be explored or understood empirically.

Consider an example of a theory about rehabilitation and interaction. The theoretic definition of the concepts are clues to the accessibility of the theory. Without definition, the words "rehabilitation" and "interaction" can assume many dimensions of meaning. If the concepts are defined, how they are to be empirically accessed is made clearer. If definitions do not clearly suggest their empiric basis and the purpose of the theory is to promote rehabilitation, an empiric basis for rehabilitation must be located within a clinical context.

Increasing the complexity within theories often increases empiric accessibility. As subconceptual categories are clarified, empiric indicators become more precise. Suppose that the concepts of rehabilitation and interaction are related within the same theory. The theory has a high degree of generality and simplicity, since the concepts are broad and few in number. Complexity can be increased by designating five subconcepts for each. Those five sub-concepts are likely to have a more precise empiric basis than the broader concepts. With empirically accessible subconcepts, the empiric accessibility of the theory increases. If a concept does not have an empiric basis at the outset, specifying subconcepts for larger wholes does not increase empiric accessibility.

Research testing establishes a foundation for determining the empiric accessibility of concepts. For example, if rehabilitation is defined operation-ally in a research project as: "attainment of 70% of full range of motion," you have established a clear link between the idea and a clinical observation. If the research supports the hypothesis derived from the theory, it also pro-vides evidence of empiric accessibility for the concept "rehabilitation."

Empiric accessibility of concepts contained within theory is basic to test-ing theoretic relationships and deliberative application of theory. Grounded approaches to generating theory assume empiric accessibility. The extent to which empiric accessibility is important can vary. Considering what the the-ory is developed to do will help you make judgments about how empirically accessible a theory should be. Theory that provides a conceptual perspective of clinical practice may not need much empiric accessibility. If a theory is to be used to guide research, empiric accessibility is important. If concepts are not empirically grounded, concept clarification may be used to provide direction for empiric indicators needed for research.

How important is this theory?

In nursing, the importance of a theory is closely tied to the idea of its clinical significance or practical value. An important theory is forward looking, use-ful, and valuable for creating a future. The central question is: "Does the theory create a reality that is important to nursing?" Many realities will be important to nursing. Some nursing theory guides research and practice, some generates radically new ideas about health and caring, and some dif-ferentiates the focus of nursing from other service professions.

If a theory contains concepts, definitions, purposes, and assumptions that are grounded in practice, it will have practical value for enhancing the-ory-based research. A theory that has limited empiric accessibility may not have practical value for research but can stimulate ideas and spark political action that improves practice.

One approach to addressing the question of importance is to reflect on the theory's basic theoretic assumptions. If underlying assumptions are unsound, the importance of the theory is minimal. If, for example, a theory is based on a view of the individual as parts, its importance for nursing is minimal. If a theory is based on an assumption of holism and it moves understanding of holism to a new dimension, it is likely to be highly important to nursing.

Theories that have extremely broad purposes may be essentially unattainable and therefore have limited value for creating clinical outcomes. This same theory may be important for generating ideas and challenging practice.

The importance of theory will depend on professional and personal values of the person who is addressing the question. Careful deliberation and discussion among nurse colleagues will help discern the importance of a theory for professional purposes.

FORMING A COMPLETE CRITICAL REFLECTION

In summary, the five questions for critically reflecting a description of theory are:

- *Is this clear?* This question addresses the clarity and consistency of presentation. Clarity and consistency may be both semantic and structural.
- *Is this simple?* This question addresses the number of structural components and relationships within theory. Complexity implies numerous relational components within theory. Simplicity implies fewer relational components.
- *Is this general?* This question addresses the scope of experiences covered by theory. Generality infers a wide scope of phenomena, whereas specificity narrows the range of events included in theory. Generality combined with simplicity yields parsimony.
- *Is this accessible?* This question addresses the extent to which concepts within the theory are grounded in empirically identifiable phenomena.
- *Is this important?* This question addresses the extent to which theory leads to valued nursing goals in practice, research, and education.

The list of questions presented in the box on pp. 138 and 139 provides a guide for forming critical reflections of theory.

CONCLUSION

The critical reflection of theory in relation to clarity, simplicity, generality, accessibility, and importance will guide the development of theory so that it is in harmony with an envisioned future. The nature of theory, as revealed with critical reflection, is basic to choosing theory for guiding research, practice, and education. In Chapter 8 we present a discussion of interrelationships between theory and research.

GUIDE FOR THE CRITICAL REFLECTION OF THEORY

How clear is this theory?

- Are major concepts defined?
- Are significant concepts not defined? Are definitions clear? Congruous? Consistent?
- Are words coined? Are coined words defined?
- Are words borrowed from other disciplines and used differently in this context?
- Is the amount of explanation appropriate? Too much? Not enough?
- Are examples or diagrams helpful? Not helpful? Needed and not present?
- Are examples and diagrams used meaningful?
- Are basic assumptions consistent with one another? With purposes?
- Is the view of person and environment compatible?
- Are the same terms defined differently?
- Are different terms defined similarly?
- Are concepts used in a manner consistent with their definition?
- Are diagrams and examples consistent with the text?
- Are compatible and coherent structures suggested for different parts of the theory?
- Can the theory be followed? Can an overall structure be diagrammed?
- Where, if any, are gaps in the flow? Do all concepts fit within the theory?
- Are there any ambiguities as a result of sequence of presentation?
- Does the theorist accomplish what she/he sets out to do?

How simple is this theory?

- How many relationships are contained within the theory?
- How are the relationships organized?
- How many concepts are contained in the theory?
- Are some concepts differentiated into subconcepts and others not?
- Can concepts be combined without losing theoretic meaning?
- Is the theory complex in some areas, not in others?
- Does the theory tend to describe, explain, or predict? Impart understanding? Create meaning?

How general is this theory?

- How specific are the purposes of this theory? Do they apply to all or only some practice areas? When?
- Is this theory specific to nursing? If not, who else could use it? Why?
- Is the purpose justifiably a nursing purpose?
- If subpurposes exist, do they reflect nursing actions? How broad are the concepts within the theory?

GUIDE FOR THE CRITICAL REFLECTION OF THEORY—cont'd.

How accessible is this theory?

- Are the concepts broad or narrow?
- How specific or general are definitions within the theory?
- Are the concepts' empiric indicators identifiable in reality? Are they within the realm of nursing?
- Do the definitions provided for the concepts adequately reflect their meanings?
- Is a very narrow definition offered for a broad concept? A broad meaning for a narrow concept?
- If words are coined, are they defined?

How important is this theory?

- Does the theory have potential to influence nursing actions? If so, to what end? Is that end desirable?
- Does the theory influence nursing education? Nursing research? If so, to what end? Is that end desirable?
- How specific are the purposes of the theory? Do they provide a general framework within which to act or a means to predict phenomena?
- Is the theory's position about people, about nursing, and about the environment consistent with nursing's philosophy?
- Given the purpose of the theory and its orientation, what of significance for nursing or health care been omitted?
- Is the stated or implied purpose one that is important to nursing? Why?
- Will use of the theory help or hinder nursing in any way? If so, how?
- Will application of this theory resolve any important issues in nursing? Will it resolve any problems?
- Is the theory futuristic and forward looking?
- Will research based on the theory answer important questions?
- Are the concepts within the domain of nursing?

REFERENCES

Ellis R: Characteristics of significant theories, Nurs Res17(3):217-222, 1968.

Fawcett J: Analysis and evaluation of conceptual models of nursing, ed 2, Philadelphia, 1989, FA Davis Co.

Hardy ME: Theories: components, development, evaluation, Nurs Res 23(2):100-107, 1974.

Stevens BJ: Nursing theory, ed 3, Boston, 1990, Little, Brown & Co.

8

Nursing theory and research

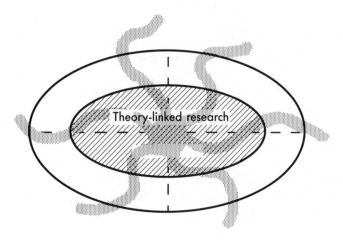

Philosophic commitments of researchers, the philosophy of
nursing, and the emerging theory are integral to the choices the
researcher makes about method. Deliberate choices that link
research methods, theory, and practice are basic to empiric
knowledge that assists nursing to achieve valued goals.

In this chapter we examine the relationship between theory and research. Although standard research texts describe the basic rules of research and the different types of research approaches that fit within these rules, the assumptions underlying the rules are not stated explicitly. Moreover, the philosophic commitments of the researcher, the fundamental philosophy of the discipline, and the theory that is emerging consistent with that philosophy are integral to the method and to choices the researcher makes about method. In this chapter we introduce ways in which research choices can be designed or evaluated to be theoretically sound.

THEORY-LINKED RESEARCH AND ISOLATED RESEARCH

Research is the systematic application of the methods of empirics in order to develop knowledge. Research can be used as a means to test theoretic relationships and as a method to generate concepts or relationships for the construction of theory.

Of all of the processes of theory development, research-related activities are more visible to the casual observer than the cognitive-based theoretic processes. The concept "research" is often associated with an image of a laboratory where experiments are conducted or where some activity occurs that involves "discovering" facts. Actually, creating empiric knowledge is more related to theory than it is to uncovering isolated facts that can be reported in great detail and numbers. Factual knowledge is useful, but facts alone are insufficient for developing empiric knowledge. In order to develop empiric knowledge, facts must be interpreted in relation to one another and conceived as having meaning (Bleich, 1978; Greer, 1969; Scheffler, 1967; Silva and Rothbart, 1984).

Research, like theorizing, can be conducted in a variety of ways and with multiple motivating factors. There are many descriptions of different types of research, and each research text presents a somewhat different way of viewing the total process. The traits of each approach that are common reflect certain basic rules that have been established in order to obtain results that are considered reliable and valid or accurately representative of empiric reality. Research problems can emerge from theories, or studies can be conducted with the intent of developing theoretic propositions. Two types of research studies are *theory-linked* and *isolated research*. The major trait that

142

distinguishes theory-linked research from isolated research is that theory-linked research is designed to develop or test theory. It is this quality that sets the stage for the study to contribute to the knowledge of the discipline. Isolated research, on the other hand, is not linked to the processes of theory development in any way.

From a research point of view, theory-linked and isolated research can both be of excellent quality. Both types of research can ultimately contribute to knowledge, although isolated research is much more limited in the contribution it can make to a discipline. Because theory-linked research is conceived and conducted within the framework of theory, the findings of research have greater potential for contributing to the development of useful knowledge.

In isolated research the investigator formulates questions or hypotheses and uses accepted methods to refute or support the hypotheses or to answer the questions. Questions or hypotheses may come from the practical circumstances surrounding the investigator's work, the imagination, an idea that occurred in reading other research results, or any number of other sources. These same factors can also provide direction for the development of theory-linked research.

Research is "done" as an activity in the empiric world and is therefore always confined to a particular place and a time in history. Since theories are constructions of the mind, they are not limited to a specific place or historical time. The cultural and historical circumstances of the theorist influence the mental construction of the theory, but, because the theory is an abstraction, it transcends the limits of particular circumstances. Isolated research, which often focuses on particulars of a specific problem, offers little potential for speculating about the significance of the research beyond that which can be justified by the method, design, and analysis of study results. Theory-linked research has advantages that overcome some of these limitations. Theory-linked research hypotheses that are developed from abstract statements of the theory represent a "translation" of the theory's abstract statements to the circumstances of the specific study. These research findings can only be generalized within limits, just as those reported in isolated research. However, the study findings in theory-linked research can be "re-translated" to theoretic terms and implications discussed in relation to the theory.

Problems of theory-linked research

Although theory-linked research has definite advantages over isolated research in being able to contribute to the development of knowledge, certain hazards and problems are unique to this type of research.

Inappropriate use of theories. It is possible to use a theory inappropriately in conducting research. For example, if a theory is designed to explain human behavior, it may not be appropriate as a basis for explaining animal behavior and vice versa. Although a theory may be considered more useful or general if it can be used to explain both animal and human behavior, it is risky to extend a theory beyond its boundaries without sufficient conceptual examination. Theory and theoretic concepts that are used inappropriately lead to erroneous conclusions. Reed (1978) describes how some theories in behavioral sciences have resulted in erroneous information concerning primate behavior. Using theories of human behavior, primate sexual behavior has been categorized as "monogamous" or "polygamous," using theories of human behavior. On the basis of limited observations of animal behavior, it became common practice to describe animal behavior using these terms. Reed points out that, in reality, animals seldom cohabitate on the basis of sex differences, and segregation of male and female primates is more pronounced than cohabitation (Reed, 1978, p. 49). Theories sometimes provide a mental set that clouds observations, especially if the theory is assumed to be "true" or consistent with prevailing values.

Theories as barriers. Theories can also obscure certain occurrences. This is because the set provided by theory, whether appropriate or not, may preclude recognition of other possibilities. When the focus is on expected outcomes, unless something startling or drastically different occurs, some elements may not be noticed. For example, you can view a child's behavior and, because of a certain theory, assume that what you observe is "problem-solving ability." Because of what the theory describes, you focus on the child's ability to manipulate objects or arrange the environment, and you call this behavior the child's ability to solve a problem. At the same time, you might fail to notice other things about the child's behavior because they are not brought to your attention by the theory. These other behaviors might include less obvious and therefore easily overlooked actions such as body posture, facial expressions, or eye motion. It is possible that qualities of these behaviors have little to do with problem-solving ability, but the mental set that you acquire from the theory focuses your attention on limited behaviors, and something potentially important in understanding the child's reality is overlooked.

Paradoxically, although a theory may be useful and appropriate for understanding reality, it may limit your thinking about the range of possibilities and experiences. Overcoming this difficulty requires that you constantly question what you read, think, and observe. Theory does not represent "truth" or "reality"; it is intended to be an approximation and a tool to see new possibilities. The purpose for using research to develop theory is to discover to what extent a theory can be regarded as sound and to what extent it functions to open new possibilities.

Ethical considerations. Theories can also exceed acceptable limits of reality; theories as mental constructions may relate ideas that cannot or should not be tested, out of respect for human and animal rights and dignity. For example, given the threat of nuclear accidents, you might imagine that it would be useful to predict events in a large population of people who experience a nuclear accident. This knowledge might help in preparing for this circumstance. In reality, it is not ethical to subject humans or animals to such an experience to develop theory. Nor is it feasible to test an "armchair" theory developed to predict the consequences of nuclear accidents.

Occasionally historical circumstances provide evidence that is used to develop useful theory, but further testing is limited by concern for human and animal welfare. Theories of mother-infant attachment and separation grew out of the experiences of wartime children separated from their mothers for extended periods of time. The evidence that grew out of the historical disaster was amply sufficient to demonstrate the harmful effects, and further research that replicates similar circumstances is ethically indefensible.

THE RELATIONSHIP BETWEEN THEORY AND RESEARCH

In this chapter our focus is on theory-linked research processes and on examining how empiric research contributes to theory development. One way of viewing this relationship between theory-linked research and theory is as a spiral (Fig. 8-1). The spiral represents the interaction between theory and research. If you begin with theory, research derived from the theory is used to clarify and extend the theory. If you begin with research, theory that is formed from the findings can be subsequently used to direct research. In order for this spiral process to continue, research must be conducted with the specific aim of contributing to theory development.

The processes of generating and testing theory, as well as deliberative application of theory, draw on research methods. Research also provides information that can be used in creating conceptual meaning and in structuring and contextualizing theory. There are essentially two ways in which research contributes to theory development: by generating theory and by testing theory.

Theory-generating research

Research that generates theory is designed to discover and describe relationships without imposing preconceived notions of what these phenomena

Theory and nursing: A systematic approach

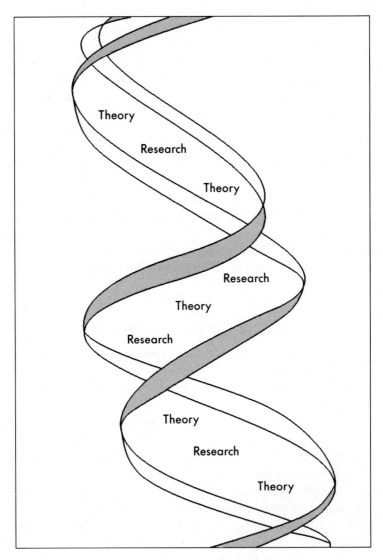

FIG. 8-1
Theory research spiral of knowledge.

mean. This is usually thought of as an inductive approach. It is impossible to observe events in the real world without some preconceived mental image of what they mean. Preexisting mental images are inherent in the experience of being socialized in a human culture; the process of learning the theories of a discipline conveys meanings. When a researcher designs a study to generate theory, observations are made with as open a mind as possible in order to see things in a new way.

As an example, suppose that a marketing analyst wanted to develop a theory about what motivates people to buy certain items. If the analyst decided to use a theory-generating approach, her research would begin by observing the shopping behavior of people in a mall. The analyst would probably already have some belief that advertising does affect behavior based on theories of behavior and marketing. Her perceptions during the observation would not be really "pure" but would be influenced by theoretic notions about how people shop. However, if the intent of the theory builder is to try to discover some previously unaccounted for variable or to describe something about shopping behavior that has not been described, preconceived ideas about this behavior must be recognized and set aside insofar as possible.

One approach to theory-generating research that has been used in nursing is grounded theory (Glaser and Strauss, 1967). This is a form of field methodology that requires the collection, coding, and categorizing of empiric observations and the formation of concepts and relationships based on the data obtained. Grounded-theory methodologies also use deductive approaches to examine propositions of theory. However, it is initially an inductive method.

Other forms of theory-generating research include field observations as used in anthropology and participant observation as used in sociology. The investigator attempts to minimize any intrusion or effect on events observed and seeks to view and describe things occurring as they would if the observer were not present. The investigator attends to clues about how one event affects another and explains the things observed by developing theoretic relationship statements about those observations (Stern, 1980).

Since many phenomena cannot be observed directly, theory-generating research must sometimes use indirect ways of gathering data. Phenomenology is one example of this approach. Phenomenology as a research method is designed to describe the subjective, lived experiences of people and to comprehend the meanings that people place on these experiences (Omery, 1983). These are experiences that cannot be observed; they are directly accessible only to the person who has the experience. Indirect ways of observing empiric reality include interviewing or questioning individuals about what they feel or remember or how they respond to certain situations. Feelings, thoughts, memories, dreams, as well as private human experiences, can only be "observed" through how people choose to relate them.

Different inductive methodologies produce different types of knowledge and different forms of descriptive statements or theories. Grounded-theory methods result in relationship statements or propositions that the researcher has observed in empiric experiences. Phenomenology results in interpretive narratives that describe meaning as fully as possible. Regardless of the approach, inductive investigators systematically organize and describe their research results.

Theory-testing research

Once theory is constructed, by whatever means, it is possible to use research methods for validation. The methods are designed to ascertain how accurately the theory depicts phenomena and their relationships. Theoretic statements can be translated into questions and hypotheses as long as the abstractions of the theory can be represented with empiric indicators. A single study is usually based on one or two relational statements from among several that might possibly be extracted from a theory. No one study can test the entirety of a theory. Some theories contain relationship statements that cannot be tested using research because empiric indicators cannot be identified.

Even though a theory has been incompletely tested, it is generally regarded as relatively sound if several research studies conducted over time in different settings tend to demonstrate a degree of confidence in the theory. If some statements tend to be supported by research, whereas others tend to be unsupported or refuted by research, the research provides a basis for revising the theory or developing new theory.

Theory-testing research is usually thought of as a deductive approach. The research starts with an abstract relational statement derived from theory. From the theoretic statement, hypotheses or research questions are created for a specific research situation.

Research questions may also be used in theory-testing research. This type of research typically uses descriptive and correlational designs. The concepts in the research questions are empirically represented, and observations are made. The data are collated and described in such a way that the questions are addressed and implications related to the development of the theory are stated.

Since hypotheses must contain a relationship between at least two variables, the research design is usually an experimental, quasi-experimental, or correlational approach (Polit and Hungler, 1987; Shelley, 1984). In theory-testing research, the investigator deliberately changes or controls conditions so that the study clearly focuses on the nature of the relationship between the variables that have been selected for study. Several descriptive and relationship testing studies are needed to eventually "test" a theory, since only a limited number from among all possible relationships can be included in one study. A single study can contribute appreciably to the validation process if it is theoretically sound.

In the following sections we examine the general research process and identify how both theory-generating and theory-testing research can be designed and therefore evaluated to achieve the most value from the research effort.

DEVELOPING SOUND THEORETIC RESEARCH

The research process can be examined for theoretic soundness at each stage. The following descriptions of each stage can serve as a guide for developing or evaluating the theoretic soundness of a research study. Examples are given in each section from two research studies to illustrate features of theory-testing and theory-generating research.

The clinical problem, research purpose, research problem, and hypotheses

In theory-linked research, the purpose, the problem statements, and the hypotheses are designed to show the relationships between the chosen theory base and the particular study being conducted. In theory-testing research, each of these statements should be explicitly formulated, for they direct movement from the broad, general intent to the empiric specifics of the study. In descriptive and exploratory theory-testing research, hypotheses may not be stated or labeled as such, and research problems (questions) are developed. Although not necessarily stated in relationship form, the questions imply underlying relationships of significance to the developing theory.

In theory-generating research only the clinical and the research problems are required; the other statements may or may not be developed explicitly in the course of the research process. These are not necessarily explicitly stated in published reports of completed research, but in well-reported studies the statements appropriate to each approach can be inferred from the text of the published article.

In theory-testing research, statements of purpose, problem, and hypotheses or questions are formulated in advance of conducting the data-gathering activity. In theory-generating research, the purpose and problem statements are formulated in advance; if relationships are stated, they are derived from the data. Table 8-1 describes the purpose served by each type of statement

TABLE 8-1

Comparison of clinical problem, research purpose, research problem, and hypothesis statements in theory-linked research

Type of statement	What the statement conveys	Theory generating*	Theory testing†
Clinical problem	Specifies the experiential observations from which the study was generated or that influenced the study Suggests the context of the study	What do nurses need to know to help women integrate menstrual care practices into their daily activities?	What factors promote health and healing?
Research purpose	Specifies whether the research is theory generating or theory testing	To generate substantive theory that explains human behavior in the social context under study.	To test Roger's principle of integrality (p. 21)
Research problem	Poses a question to be answered Is less general than the purpose and makes clear how the purpose is to be achieved Expresses the nature of the variable or events to be studied Implies the empiric possibilities for the abstract concepts given in the purpose Expresses the relationships between concepts if the relationship is the focus for the study	How do women integrate menstrual care practices into daily activities? (p. 19)	How do changes in environmental resonance change a person's perception of rest? (p. 22)
Hypothesis	Indicates the specific choices made in relation to the variables for the study Implies the design of the study Implies the type of analysis used	The making-sure process is comprised of three subprocesses: (1) attending, (2) calculating, and (3) juggling (p. 25). (generated from the study data)	The perception of restfulness will be lower (subjects more rested) for confined subjects who experience varied harmonious auditory input than for those who experience quiet ambience (p. 23).

*Examples are from Patterson ET and Hale ES: Making sure: integrating menstrual care practices into activities of daily living, Adv Nurs Sci 7(3):18-31, 1985.
†Examples are from Smith, MJ: Human-environment process: a test of Rogers' principle of integrality. Adv Nurs Sci 9(1):21-28, 1986.

and shows how clinical problem, research purpose, research problem, and hypotheses follow from each other and provide a conceptual link between the theory and the research study.

As the table shows, there are two types of problems: clinical and research. The clinical problem is a question that reflects the general experiential concern that generated or influenced the study and suggests the study context. The clinical problem does not specify or imply relationships but simply indicates the context within which theoretic relationships will be generated or tested.

The research purpose indicates whether the study is theory generating or theory testing in nature and whether the study focuses on description, explanation, or prediction. If the study is for the purpose of generating theory, the purpose further states the empiric reality the investigator is studying. If the study is theory testing, the purpose states the theoretic frame of reference for the study.

For both theory-generating and theory-testing research, the research problem is less general than the statement of purpose and directs the more specific, circumstantial focus of the study. The research problem is phrased in the form of a question. The question implies how the purpose of the study is to be achieved. It reflects the variables or events to be studied and implies that empiric possibilities for abstract concepts to be developed are embodied in existing theoretic relationships.

When hypotheses are stated, they indicate the circumstantial restrictions of the study . Hypotheses should also reflect the study design and suggest the analysis to be made of data. Hypotheses usually provide specific guidance for statistical analysis of qualitative data. If the analysis of the research data does not depend on statistics for drawing conclusions, hypotheses might not be stated.

In theory-generating research hypotheses may or may not be stated. Problem statements or research questions may be appropriate for guiding a study intended to generate theory, and hypotheses are formulated at the conclusion of the study, if at all. When formulated, hypotheses provide specific direction for future research.

Background of the study and literature review

In all research the literature review surveys research findings that are pertinent to the study being conducted. In theory-linked research the literature review also includes a summary evaluation of the theoretic background for the study.

For theory-generating research the background for the study includes a review of previous writings, including the theoretic, philosophic, and empiric studies pertinent to the area of concern. The author's thinking and experience are important as background for the study. The literature review is not necessarily completed in advance. As the ideas and concepts emerge from the data, the researcher uses the data to guide explorations in the existing literature. The empiric observations remain the primary source for analysis and interpretation, but in some instances the literature provides a basis for refining and delineating central concepts and the relationships between them.

In theory-testing research, previous studies based on the theory form a substantial portion of the literature review. The review also contains a critique of previous research based on alternative theories and on concepts or variables shown to be related to the study's central purpose. The review traces how the study has been conceived and summarizes the theoretic ideas that are being tested. This clarifies how and why specific relationships within the theory are being tested.

In Table 8-1, Smith's study (1986) is used to show how statements of clinical problem, research purpose, research problem, and hypotheses are formulated. In this study report, the background includes a description of the portion of Martha Rogers' theoretic framework that formed the basis for study. The background focuses on explaining the way in which the study variable "rest" was conceptualized. The related literature provided evidence that substantiated the author's conceptualization. "Rest" in this study was conceptualized as "the person's experience of easing with the flow of rhythmic change in the environment . . . [reflecting] person and environment as open systems in ever-changing integral interplay with each other." The auditory environment was the environmental field that was selected for specific focus in this study.

Patterson and Hale's report of grounded theory (one approach to theory-generating research) (1985, p. 25) illustrates the conception of a research idea from questioning traditional notions about limiting the levels of activity for menstruating women. The literature they reviewed substantiated that, historically, attitudes toward menstruation have remained negative. Because the authors were interested in the significance of their question for nursing practice, they reviewed Orem's self-care theory, noting the importance of translating self-care concepts to several domains of nursing practice. As is typical in theory-generating research, the authors cite a void in research related to how women manage their menstrual flow. The authors also point out that research on menstruation has focused on medical problems, that is, dysmenorrhea and premenstrual distress. From Patterson and Hale's perspective, this existing literature on menstruation offers no background for building and influencing the development of concepts and theoretic relationships significant to nursing. However, Orem's theory does provide a basis for later development of relationships.

The research method

Several concerns with regard to research method must be carefully considered when theory-linked research is undertaken. These include the means of obtaining the data, the selection of the sample for study, the design of the research, and the analysis of data and conclusions.

The means of obtaining data. How the data are collected or recorded must be consistent with the purpose of the research design. For theory-generating research, the study is usually descriptive in nature and requires either direct or indirect observation and recording of empiric events that the investigator does not alter or change during the course of study. Theory-testing research also draws on these means of obtaining data. Because this type of research often relies on some type of experimental or correlation analysis, the tools used tend to be those that yield quantitative measures of the variables.

Direct observation requires being physically present. Data are recorded by some means, such as note-taking or audio or video taping. Examples include watching and making notations about behavior during the processes of mother-infant bonding, interactions between nurses and clients within an intensive care unit, or behavior of a person experiencing a crisis such as pain.

Indirect observation includes the following: interviewing; using questionnaires and standardized tools that elicit feelings, thoughts, memories; or self-reports of experiences not directly observable. Tools designed to elicit reports about selected phenomena must be carefully examined to be sure they can provide the evidence needed to achieve the purposes of the study. Tools developed with a particular theoretic basis introduce a perspective that may not be desirable in theory-generating research. Paradoxically, a tool developed to explore several possibilities regarding the reality of an experience may be needed for theory-generating research, yet may lack the reliability and validity needed for accurate results. In theory-testing research the means of obtaining data must be carefully considered in relation to theoretic adequacy of tools and measurement approaches. In both types of research, the problems of reliability and validity of both direct and indirect observations are considered. Tools that are designed to yield a numeric score are assessed for reliability and validity using the methods of statistics. Tools and interview approaches that are designed to produce narrative descriptions are examined carefully to ascertain how well the approach will function to elicit the type of responses that are needed. The research report should include a discussion of the level of development for the tools used, what theoretic perspective underlies any tools used, and what evidence exists of the tool's reliability and validity.

In Smith's study (1986), Borg's tool of perceived exertion was modified to form a tool of perceived restfulness. The author discusses research evidence that supports the reliability and validity of the Borg tool, the modifications she made to develop the tool, and the results of her own preliminary findings regarding the reliability and validity of the modified tool. In addition she discusses issues concerning the measurement of fatigue and energy levels and the approaches that other researchers have taken. She concludes that it is reasonable to measure energy levels by asking people to express differences in their experiences of energy.

In Patterson and Hale's study of menstrual care practices, interviews were the primary method for obtaining data, because social norms dictate that menstruation be concealed. Other methods for obtaining data included anecdotes shared by friends; serendipitous, informal observations (e.g., conversations in restrooms, advertisements); and personal menstrual experience.

The selection of the sample. The selection of the sample is essentially what limits the research to a particular time and place. It is a part of the research that links the abstractions of the theory with empiric phenomena. In theory-generating research the investigator alleges, "There is some phenomenon or event happening in reality that will be evident if I observe this particular group of people. Furthermore, this particular group is sufficiently like other groups of people who have this experience to represent them." The individuals chosen for the sample are purposely selected because they can contribute information and insight related to the phenomenon being studied.

In theory-testing research, sample selection requires the investigator to take the position that, if the theory being tested is empirically reasonable, it will be supported by what happens with the specific persons selected for study. Or, if the theory is not empirically accurate, the responses of the sample studied will refute the theory. Since most theory-testing research relies on statistical analysis of quantitative data, sample selection is guided by the requirements of statistical analysis. Both the population to whom the theoretic relationship applies and the sample that is being tested must be specified. Drawing the conclusion of empiric accuracy of the relationship depends on being able to assume that the statistical requirements for sampling from the identified population have been met.

In Patterson and Hale's study of menstrual care activities, sample selection was guided by the type of theory that was being developed. Initially the investigators approached healthy women living in the community. As the theory began to emerge, other healthy women in the community were identified and invited to participate because of life experiences the investigators were beginning to consider as theoretically relevant. For example, a lawyer was included because her work demands were intense and often interfered with menstrual care activities.

In the report of Smith's theory-testing study, the sample consisted of 60 men and 60 women who considered themselves to be healthy and who were between the ages of 18 and 35. They were all volunteers and were randomly assigned to one of the two study groups. The criterion for sample selection was consistent with Rogers' theory (1970) on which the study was based; that is, persons included had to be healthy (no known health problems) and willing to participate in the study.

The research design. The design of the research outlines the procedure and contingencies used for answering the research questions or testing the hypotheses. In theory-generating research, the design must be consistent with the theory-generating orientation of the research. This often involves observation of a particular kind of phenomenon of interest in given groups. Stern (1980) describes the design of grounded theory as a matrix in which several research processes are in operation at once. The investigator examines the data as obtained and begins to code, categorize, conceptualize, and write impressions about its meaning.

Sometimes research designs that are typically used in theory-testing research are needed for theory-generating research. This is the case when a sequence of ordinarily occurring events is an area of concern. For example, suppose something happens to create a sequence of events, such as the birth of a child or the death of a loved one. The research interest might be to describe the usual responses of individuals over a period of time, both before and after this event, in order to generate theory regarding how people react in these situations. In these instances comparative assessments over time are needed. The investigator does not, as in classic experimental designs, impose the changes as a part of the design but rather waits for the changes to occur. The investigator then describes the nature of outcomes occurring before and after the event in order to develop theory.

Theory-generating research also may require comparison groups that are typical of experimental designs in order to determine if a phenomenon occurs only under certain circumstances. Suppose, for example, that an investigator wanted to determine if body image formation were appreciably affected by chronic illness. The phenomenon could be studied by comparing body image formation in a group of people having a chronic illness with body image formation in a group not having chronic illness. The comparison would determine if aspects of the phenomenon "body image formation" were unique to people with chronic illness. This information would contribute to the development of theory related to body image formation.

In some forms of theory-testing research, the researcher deliberately alters circumstances in some way in order to test the relationships expressed in the hypotheses. The design usually includes some intervention or investigator-created circumstances consistent with the theoretic basis for the study.

In Smith's theory testing study (1986), a two-group pretest-posttest experimental design was used to test the effects of auditory input on perceptions of restfulness. The researcher designed a laboratory environment where the participants could rest on a bed for 150 minutes in a controlled auditory environment and complete the perceived restfulness tool before and after the specified period of rest while being observed through a one-way mirror. One group was provided a quiet auditory environment, which consisted of a non-speaking, hushed environment in which only sporadic muffled sounds could be heard. The experimental group was provided a carefully designed and controlled sequence of auditory input that alternated between music, silence, story, silence, music, silence, story, silence, and music.

In Patterson and Hale's study of menstrual care practices, a grounded-theory approach was selected for two reasons—because criticism in the literature reflected a lack of fit between theory and practice in studying women's experience in general, and because there was a need to accurately conceptualize phenomena that occur within the nursing domain (Patterson and Hale, 1985, p. 21) The grounded-theory approach provides a continuous and interactive process that promotes a fit between what women actually experience and the theory that emerges as a result of coding that experience. This approach also provides for conceptualizing a phenomenon that is clearly within nursing's domain but that had not been previously described in the literature.

Analysis of the data and conclusions. The analysis of data in theory-linked research must be consistent with the purposes of the research and the research design. For theory-generating research, analysis of data involves narrative, descriptive, and other relatively qualitative types of analysis. Depending on the type of observation used, a quantitative, numeric, or statistical analysis of the data can also be presented, but this is accompanied by a theoretic analysis that includes the full range of observations and the ways in which the observations occurred.

In a grounded-theory approach, analysis of the data involves coding and categorizing the observations. In participant observation the analysis may report sample observations that typify the characteristic events or the sequence of events that was observed. Whatever the form of data presentation, the investigator proposes concepts generated from the data and, if possible, a description of theoretic propositions that emerge from the data. The extent to which concepts and theoretic propositions are formulated depends on how well the evidence supports making conceptual and theoretic formulations, as well as the extent to which previous studies support such conceptual and theoretic development.

In theory-testing research, analysis of the data should present sufficient quantitative and qualitative evidence to support or reject the hypotheses or to address the research questions. The conclusions of the study should include an interpretive analysis of the findings in relation to the theory being tested. The analysis of data focuses on the specific study findings, whereas the conclusions focus on the theoretic significance of the study.

In Patterson and Hale's grounded-theory method, the data analysis involved coding transcriptions from taped interviews and other incidents, collapsing the codes into higher level concepts, writing theoretic ideas sparked by the coding, and drawing relationships between concepts. In the report, quotes from the transcription were used to substantiate the results of coding and sorting. The process of data analysis led to the following summary of the substantive process:

> The making-sure process is comprised of three subprocesses: (1) attending, (2) calculating, and (3) juggling. These states of making sure are analogous to Orem's types of self-care operations—estimative, transitional, and productive—and provide substantive elaboration on these concepts. Estimative operations are oriented to the individuals making judgments about what is, transitional operations end in a determination of what should be done, and production operations are the regulatory activities (p. 25).

Patterson and Hale's conclusion addresses further theory development in relation to recurrent self-care operations, particularly those required for other involuntary eliminative phenomena such as that experienced by someone with an ostomy. Suggestions for nursing practice and for further research are given on the basis of the study findings.

In Smith's theory testing study (1986), numeric data from the pretest and postest scores were presented, as well as the results of statistical analyses of differences between the experimental and the control groups on the scores of perceived restfulness. Results indicated that the group who received varied auditory input were more rested than the group who received a hushed auditory environment. This finding supported the research hypothesis of the study. In discussing this finding, the author explained the implications concerning the theoretic ideas on which the study was based. Her conclusion stated:

> This [the finding that harmonic auditory input is effective in promoting restfulness] contributes support to the principle of integrality in that it demonstrates that the human-environment field process is continuous; that is, the human field and the environmental field are mutually integrated (p. 27).

Generalizability and usefulness of the study

In theory-linked research, one of the important considerations for a single study is how this particular study contributes to theory development. In most instances a single study raises more questions that it answers, and questions raised must be presented in order to provide a basis for future study. Theory-generating research should evolve relationship statements that can be studied and used in further developing the theory. Theory-testing research may result in evidence that suggests revision or extension of the theory tested, or it may suggest an entirely new avenue for development of theory.

Theory-generating research is often immediately useful for practice. Theory-testing research can also have immediate practice application. If the research design is valid and the findings are generalizable and consistent with related research findings, the investigator may conclude that certain approaches in the realm of practice might be useful. However, immediate use in practice cannot always be expected. The primary value of theory-testing research is to stimulate further study and theory development that will add to empiric knowledge on which practice can be based.

CONCLUSION

Theory-linked research may be either theory-generating or theory-testing. Research approaches can be used to test theoretic relationships and in formal application of theory and can contribute to the structuring of theoretic relationships. Links between research and theory are basic to empiric knowledge that assists in achieving valued nursing goals. In Chapter 9 we consider the relationships between theory and practice.

REFERENCES

Bleich D: Subjective criticism, Baltimore, 1978, Johns Hopkins University Press.

Campbell DT and Stanley JC: Experimental and quasi-experimental designs for research, Chicago, 1963, Rand McNally & Co.

Glaser B and Strauss A: The discovery of grounded theory, Chicago, 1967, Aldine Publishing Co.

Greer S: The logic of social inquiry, Chicago, 1969, Aldine Publishing Co.

Omery A: Phenomenology: a method for nursing research, Adv Nurs Sci 5(2):63, 1983.

Patterson ET and Hale ES: Making sure: integrating menstrual care practices into activities of daily living, Adv Nurs Sci 7(3):18-31, 1985.

Polit B and Hungler B: Nursing research, ed 3, Philadelphia, 1987, JB Lippincott Co.

Reed E: Sexism and science, New York, 1978, Pathfinder Press.

Rogers ME: An introduction to the theoretical basis of nursing, Philadelphia, 1970, FA Davis Co.

Scheffler I: Science and subjectivity, Indianapolis, 1967, The Bobbs-Merrill Company, Inc.

Shelley, SI: Research methods in nursing and health, Boston, 1984, Little, Brown & Co.

Silva MC and Rothbart D: An analysis of changing trends in philosophies of science on nursing theory development and testing, Adv Nurs Sci 6(2):1-13, 1984.

Smith MJ: Human environment process: A test of Roger's principle of integrality, Adv Nurs Sci 9(1):21-28, 1986.

Stern PN: Grounded theory methodology: its uses and processes, Image 12(1):20-23, 1980.

9

Nursing theory and practice

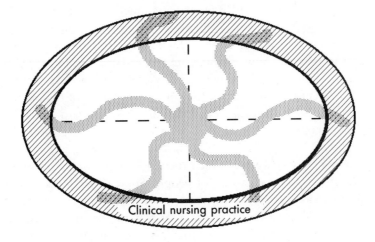

Clinical nursing practice

If theory is expected to benefit practice, it must be developed cooperatively with people who practice nursing. People who do research and develop theories think differently about theory when they perceive the reality of practice.

If theory is expected to benefit practice, it must be developed cooperatively with people who practice nursing. There are important relationships between nursing practice and the processes of theory development. Theories do not provide the same type of procedural guidelines for practice as do situation-specific principles and procedures or rules (Beckstrand, 1980). Procedural rules or principles help to standardize nursing practice and can be useful in achieving minimum goals of quality of care. Theories exist to challenge existing practice, create new approaches to practice, and remodel the structure of rules and principles.

One way that theory challenges existing practice is that it provides new ways to think about problems. Thinking about a problem or a situation in a new or different way makes it possible for practitioners to envision new approaches to practice. Since theories are not sets of rules, but are tentative, practice also challenges theory. The processes of theory development as described in Chapter 5 depend on the continual "tests" of the practice perspective. People who do research and develop theories learn to think differently about theoretic problems and issues as they perceive the realities of practice.

By *nursing practice* we mean the experiences a practicing nurse encounters during the process of caring for people. Some experiences are those of the client, others are those of the nurse, some are interactive, and some are environmental. These experiences may also occur in other settings, but, when they occur in the context of providing nursing care, they are considered part of nursing practice.

In this chapter we address specific ways in which practitioners can contribute to theory development processes. One avenue is through the process of creating conceptual meaning, which brings together the practical and the theoretic to benefit both practitioner and theorist. The deliberative application of theory also provides specific opportunities for practicing nurses to make critical decisions regarding when and how to apply theory in practice and how to judge the effect of the theory's application on the broader goals of nursing practice. Although nurses use theory in practice in many different ways, in this chapter we consider how practice contributes to and benefits from processes of creating conceptual meaning and deliberative application of entire theories.

CREATING CONCEPTUAL MEANING

Concepts do not simply appear or arise; they develop from perceived experience. The perceptual experiences from which nursing concepts develop are found in the practice of nursing. Practicing nurses who reflect on the nature of their experiences make significant contributions to theory development. Individuals who are primarily involved in theory development benefit from the ideas of many nurses who practice nursing. Individuals do not participate equally in all processes required for the development of theory; rather, it is a collective endeavor.

Empiric concepts are formed from nursing practice by observing, naming, and making sense of what happens there. A concept is not the experience itself. The mental image that develops from the experience and the language that is used to convey the idea make it possible for practitioners and others to communicate about that experience. Concepts are generally ambiguous, particularly to an experienced practitioner who prefers precise guides for practice. But, even with ambiguity, concepts provide a mental tool for quickly comprehending a range of specific experiences and thinking about what those experiences mean. Once concepts are integrated into theory, the theory provides explanations that bring to awareness interpretations of specific situations.

The processes of creating conceptual meaning (described in Chapter 5) can be used as ways to draw on experiences in nursing practice that contribute to theory development. One approach is to present practice situations as model, related, or borderline cases for concepts. The practice situation is also useful for identifying appropriate empiric indicators for nursing concepts. The following sections describe four practice-dependent activities that contribute to the process of theory development in nursing.

Identification of empiric indicators

Practice provides essential evidence that is used to select empiric indicators for abstract concepts. The experiences of practice can challenge existing theoretic conceptualizations, and they can reveal hunches that have not yet been linked to a particular concept or theory. The basic question is: "What have I experienced that can be linked to the abstract concept 'X'?" (anxiety, for example).

Suppose that a wide range of behaviors observed in practice are described in a theory as manifestations of the concept "anxiety." These behaviors might include wringing of hands, silence and refusal to talk, excessive talking, laughter, crying, sweating, compulsive eating, or lack of appetite. Tools have been constructed that measure the concept using these empiric indicators. In your practice experience, you observe that these ideas do not always "fit." When you work with individuals who are anxious, you observe that they tend to behave in ways that are not consistent with the theoretic concept. There are some behaviors that you almost never observe and others that are commonly experienced but not taken into account by the theory. Since anxiety as an abstract idea does convey something that you know exists, it might be helpful if you could better identify it, understand how it works, and determine how people experience it differently. As you draw on your experience, new ideas begin to emerge from the empiric behaviors you have noticed. This information is invaluable for the practice-sensitive theorist.

Differentiating similar concepts

Concepts that are similar yet different might share certain empiric indicators, and differentiating them from one another may be difficult. If knowing the difference between them is important in practice, practice can provide the empiric information and conceptual insights required to distinguish one from another. This purpose becomes critical when you realize that errors can be made in assigning meaning to a person's experience. For example, you might have been taught that certain behaviors are manifestations of anxiety, based on a popular theory of anxiety. You have developed an approach to assist people who are anxious to reduce their anxiety and improve their function, but it does not seem to be as effective as you think it should be. One problem might be that the behaviors are not indicative of anxiety, but are associated with another feeling. Your challenge is to begin to conceptualize anxiety more clearly, conceptualize what else might be happening, and begin to find ways to differentiate between the two or more experiences. As you question and challenge the conceptualization and the conclusions that you draw from it, you will form a basis for restructuring the concepts and form new or revised concepts that better represent nursing experience.

Model cases and related cases drawn from practice are extremely valuable to differentiate between similar experiences. This involves a considerable degree of flexibility in thinking. A case that initially appears to represent one type of experience may become less clearly a model case as you consider closely related cases. Gradually you will form ideas that reveal essential similarities and differences between the closely related experiences. These ideas can be integrated into the criteria for the concepts. As an example, Table 9-1 lists criteria to differentiate the concept "empathy" from the related concepts of "sympathy," "pity," and "compassion" (Forsyth, 1980). Three criteria for all instances of related concepts are also criteria for empathy: con-

TABLE 9-1
Criteria for empathy and related concepts*

Provisional criteria	Empathy	Sympathy	Pity	Compassion
Consciousness	X	X	X	X
Temporality	X	X	X	X
"I-thou" relationship	X			
Validation	X			
Accuracy	X			
Intensity	X	X	X	X
Objectivity	X			
Subjectivity		X	X	X
Freedom from value judgment	X			

*Modified from Forsyth, GL Analysis of the concept of empathy: illustration of one approach, Adv Nurs Sci 2 (2):40, 1980. Used with permission of Aspen Systems Corporation.

sciousness, temporality, and intensity. Subjectivity, a criterion for all the related concepts, is not a criterion for empathy. Further, five additional criteria are required for empathy that are not required for instances of related concepts.

Identification of new concepts

Creating conceptual meaning is a process that can lead to the identification of new concepts. Model, borderline, related, and contrary cases that come from practice reflect the richness and complexity of practice. As you reflect deliberately on these situations, your insights can lead to new ideas that contribute to forming new concepts.

For example, suppose you begin to notice that there is something about how people learn in the postoperative period that does not seem to be described in any of the literature you have read. Most learning theories have been developed and tested within classroom or laboratory settings where learners are students or other types of "healthy" subjects. In nursing situations, the learner is often experiencing an altered health state, and the patterns of behavior that are the focus of learning in this context have not been addressed in developing concepts and theories of learning. As you reflect on your experience, you see meanings that are different from the meaning of learning in the existing learning theories. As you discuss your ideas with other nurses, you find that they have made similar observations. From this awareness you can build a new conceptualization that, once named, can be incorporated into theory and used in practice.

Identification of criteria for nursing diagnoses

Although criteria for nursing diagnoses are not the same as criteria for a concept as used in theory development, nursing diagnostic criteria can be derived partially from criteria for a concept. Nursing diagnostic criteria take into account generally accepted standards for practice, as well as knowledge and application of many areas of theory that are pertinent to the diagnosis. Consider, for example, the nursing diagnosis, "Altered parenting related to impaired parental-infant attachment." In practice, the purpose is to accurately identify when this occurs in order to provide effective nursing care. The phrase "impaired parental-infant attachment" implies knowledge of human attachment theory and also suggests the focus for nursing actions. The phrase "altered parenting" implies that knowledge of the concept of parenting is required—a concept less well developed in the empiric realm than are theories of attachment. When criteria for nursing diagnoses are derived in part from a concept not yet well developed, the process of creating conceptual meaning can be used to form tentative diagnostic criteria that can be tested for empiric accuracy or validity.

The criteria for the nursing diagnosis of "altered parenting related to impaired parental-infant attachment" could include conceptual criteria for parenting. The diagnostic criteria also include value qualifiers such as the term "altered" that conveys the value that the practitioner assigns to a situation in the process of making clinical decisions. When the parent being considered is the mother, the diagnostic criteria might be:

- Visual contact between mother and infant is minimal or absent.
- Physical touching of the infant by the mother is limited to necessary touch.
- There is minimal or no vocalization by the mother directed to the infant.
- The mother's verbal expressions focus on herself (that is, concerns for her own body or image or relationships with peers, rather than expressions focusing on the infant).
- Care of the infant resembles doll play and is easily or passively given over to another caretaker.

These diagnostic criteria do not include all conceptual criteria for "mothering" that are given as an example in Chapter 5, but they do reflect how one set of criteria for practice relates to another set of criteria for theory development. The choice of diagnostic criteria focuses on those that can be empirically observed and measured in practice. The diagnostic criteria may or may not be sufficient to use in formal testing of the theoretic concept. Evidence of the diagnostic criteria recorded in practice does provide a basis for decisions about how research should proceed. If the purpose of creating conceptual meaning is to form criteria useful for nursing diagnosis, then traits that are observed in practice and that can be verified and assessed need to be emphasized.

DELIBERATIVE APPLICATION OF THEORY

Deliberative application of theory involves using research methods to demonstrate how a theory affects nursing practice. Deliberative application of theory places theory within the context of practice to ensure that it serves the goals of the profession. Deliberative application provides evidence of the theory's usefulness in ensuring quality of care.

Deliberative application of theory is the essence of the theory-practice relationship. Theory that addresses goals of practice provides a way to systematically develop substantial empiric knowledge within the discipline. Theory is not a quick and easy answer to a problem but rather provides knowledge and understanding to ultimately enhance the practice of nursing.

A first step is to ascertain if the theory can be applied in practice. Some theories that hold promise may not be sufficiently developed to justify their application. Others might be poorly suited to a particular practice area. The guidelines we suggest in the following section can be used to make this decision. Once you decide to apply the theory in practice, you can then design research methods to demonstrate how well the theory contributes to your practice goals through the deliberative application of theory.

HOW TO DETERMINE IF A THEORY SHOULD BE APPLIED IN PRACTICE

We have stated that theory ought to ultimately improve nursing practice. Usually this goal is achieved by using theory or portions of theory to guide practice. We have also cautioned against the misuse of theory in practice, and most nursing scholars lament premature or uninformed application of theory. These cautions are well founded, and it is important to consider how sound judgments regarding the application of theory in practice are made.

One of the most common ways theory has been organized for practice is in the nursing process of analyzing assessment data. Sometimes this is termed the "scientific rationale for designing nursing care plans." In practice, judgments are often made without conscious effort or explicit explanation of the basis for the judgment. If called upon to do so, most nurses could cite some valid reasons for their judgments. Although the theories cited may provide an explanation that seems rational and well founded, it is important to seriously consider how adequate the theories are as a basis for making judgments. The adequacy of theories is equally critical when they are considered as a basis for directing nursing actions.

Theory is not the only means by which nursing practice can improve, nor does theory provide the only possible basis for practice. Certain common practices in nursing have emerged from sound principles or standards based in fundamental truths that have not yet come under sufficient challenge to be a focus for theory development. As Beckstrand (1980, p. 73) has noted, "Principles of practice are shorthand ways of referring to fundamental truths to be considered and general customs to be followed." Standards of practice reflect valued actions that are generally accepted in a given situation. Principles and standards are judged by their consistent outcomes; for example, do they consistently yield desired results in practice? They are changed not by systematically challenging the standards or the principles themselves but rather by discovering another approach that better achieves the desired outcome (Beckstrand, 1980).

Theory, in contrast, cannot be assumed to predict a desired outcome and does not exist to give specific guidelines for what "should" be done in a given situation. Rather, theory predicts a possible relationship that can be questioned. The goal of the theory and the goals of practice should be consistent with one another, but this cannot be assumed to be the case. If the relationships predicted by the theory are faulty or do not accurately represent reality, the theory may not be effective in achieving practice goals. Theory can be effectively used to describe, explain, and predict a phenomenon that occurs in practice, but may not adequately contribute to the goals of practice if it is applied. Since any application of theory will affect practice, deliberative use of theory cannot be undertaken lightly. The questions we suggest in the following section can be used to reach an informed decision about application of the theory so that its practice value can be assessed.

Are the theory goals and practice goals congruous with one another?

To answer this question, examine the goal of the theory and compare it with the outcomes or goals that you see as valuable for nursing practice. The existing standards of practice can be used as one basis for clarifying the values upon which your practice is based and the overall goals that your practice should be reflecting. Another basis for identifying practice goals is your own view of nursing and that of nurses with whom you work. If a theoretic goal would lead to a situation that is not congruous with your idea of optimal health, for example, the theory may not be one that you would want to use.

Sometimes this judgment is not easily accomplished and requires a deliberate philosophic stance with regard to nursing, health, the individual, and society. For example, application of a theory may be undertaken to determine if the theoretic goal is consistent with the goal of optimal health. If the theoretic goal is adaptation and if this concept is not consistent with your idea of optimal health, you would not use a theory of adaptation in your practice.

Is the intended context of the theory congruous with the situation in which the theory will be applied?

This question addresses how well suited the theory is for your situation, given the general ideas of context that are stated or implied theoretically. A theory of pain alleviation, for example, may explain the processes involved in alleviating pain in any instance in which it occurs. As you become familiar with the theory, you realize that it was developed with reference to mature adults, and you work with children. You and your colleagues would need to explore how well the ideas of the theory might transfer to your own situation before you make a decision to proceed with application of the theory.

Is there, or might there be, similarity between theory variables and practice variables?

This question compares the important variables in the construction of the theory with the variables recognized to be directly influencing the practice situation. In some instances important practice variables may not be included in the theoretic relationship statements. For example, a learning theory may not consider the health status of the learner, and the learner is assumed to be a healthy individual. If practice variables are not accounted for in the theory or if there are substantial differences between the theoretic variables and the practice variables, the theory should be applied with caution, if at all. If the theory appears to have value and satisfies the considerations of most people who will be involved in the deliberative application process, it might be applied with systematic observation of the effect on outcomes, considering the differing variables that occur in practice.

Are the explanations of the theory sufficient to be used as a basis for nursing action?

Responses to this question must be based on expert judgment about the particular nursing actions that are implied within the theory. As an expert nurse, you may find it difficult to describe the basis on which you would judge a theory to be sufficient or not sufficient. One specific approach in forming your ideas is to examine the correspondence between theoretic and practice variables. If variables in the nursing situation are similar to those that are suggested in the theory, you can then consider the nature of the relationships between the concepts of the theory. Examine the extent to which the explanation makes sense, in light of your practice. You may feel guarded about the "sense" of the theory for practice, but can see that the perspective of the theory is reasonable. In this case, the theory is probably sufficient as a basis for nursing action, but your tentativeness about it leads you to be appropriately cautious as you proceed to use it.

An example of a sufficient theoretic explanation for application in practice is that of attachment theory. Hospitalization of children has created a classic separation response in those children who are separated from their significant parent. The theory describes behaviors (variables) that are clearly observed in hospitalized children. The theory also provides explanations for this phenomenon and predictions about the effects of severe or prolonged separation. Moreover, predictions are made concerning healthy outcomes that could be expected if child and parent separation were made less intense or prolonged. The theory provides direction for the nursing actions that are needed. These are not exact actions or specific rules or principles, but the theory does suggest types of actions that reduce separation and promote attachment.

Is there research evidence supporting the theory?

One very influential source of information for deciding whether or not a theory can be applied in practice is research evidence. Sometimes a theorist, in presenting the theory, provides research evidence to support the initial theoretic formulation. If the evidence is convincing and attracts sufficient attention in the discipline, the professional literature will report research that either validates the initial theoretic relationships or does not support the theory. Research reports often suggest limits on the range of applicability of the theory or flaws in the initial theoretic construction based on the research evidence generated.

Since few theories are unequivocally supported by research evidence, it is the responsibility of the practitioners to determine if the evidence is sufficient to justify application of the theory in practice. This judgment is best made on the basis of several research studies. If there is little or no research evidence to justify application in practice, but most of the other concerns have been satisfied, you can feel reasonably comfortable about applying the theory. In this case you should give particular attention to observing and recording relevant information regarding corresponding theoretic and situational variables and the limits and outcomes of the theory's application in practice.

How will this new approach influence the practical function of the nursing unit?

Before applying a theory in practice, you need to consider the ways in which this approach will affect the functioning of the nursing unit and assess the potential for observing and recording factors that are relevant to the theory's application. Successful application will depend on planning for the changes that are required, including the changes that will be needed to gather the research data for deliberative application. Questions to be addressed in planning for application include:

- Do nursing personnel need to be oriented to the theory and its application?
- Does the approach require adjustments in the function or processes of the nursing unit?
- Does the approach require additional time or an adjustment in the allocation of time?
- Will the approach require new equipment or other material resources?
- What practical arrangements and materials are needed to enhance the ease and accuracy of making and recording observations?
- How will trial application affect other activities in the setting?
- Are special provisions needed for gathering and storing information?
- How will clients be informed regarding the approaches that will be used?
- How will the data that are obtained be assessed and analyzed?
- If the theoretic goal is attained or not attained, how will the results be explained or accounted for?
- Have alternative explanations been projected in order to have sufficient information to make a judgment about outcomes?
- How will the results of the experience be compiled in order to communicate them to others?

If each of these questions can be answered in such a way that application seems feasible and desirable, application is probably indicated.

QUALITY-RELATED OUTCOMES

Methods that are used in the deliberative application of theory are drawn from the methods of evaluation research (Schroeder, 1984; Smeltzer, Hinshaw, and Feltman, 1987). These methods depend on knowing what outcomes you wish to achieve and on having a well-planned approach for achieving the goal. In deliberative application of theory, the approach is the application of a selected theory in a particular practice situation, as described in the previous section. The evaluation research methods depend on having some means for determining what circumstances exist prior to the application and comparing this with the results following the application. Usually factors associated with the outcomes are identified and measured before beginning and again after the approach has been in place for a specified period of time. The following sections describe quality-related outcomes that you might consider in planning deliberative application.

Professional standards of care

The standards of nursing practice that are accepted by the nursing practice unit can be the measure for assessing outcomes related to deliberative application of theory. Since standards of care often reflect minimum acceptable practice, you may consider what extensions of the standards might be desirable in assessing the effects of the theory's application on the quality of nursing practice.

Functional outcomes

Nursing goals are sometimes defined in terms of how efficiently the work of nursing is done, how cost-effective it is, or how smoothly the work of each individual coordinates with the work of others. If these factors have been identified as a problem for a particular unit, the factors that are indicative of the problem need to be clearly specified and assessed prior to applying theory. Once the baseline data are obtained and the approach based on the theory has been in place for a period of time, the measures of functional effectiveness are obtained and compared.

Nurse satisfaction

Satisfaction with respect to nursing job responsibilities can be closely related to functional outcomes. Nurse job satisfaction can be assessed by such factors as working conditions, relationships with colleagues, personal fulfillment, various types of perceived benefits, or perceived dissatisfactions. A premise underlying the selection of this type of outcome is that, if nurses are satisfied with their work situation, the quality of care they provide will improve.

Quality of care perceived by the person who receives care

People who receive care can be interviewed to ascertain their perception of the quality of care. There are several aspects of perceived quality of care that can be measured, including satisfaction with specific dimensions of care, perceived benefits from the care, and perceived dissatisfactions.

Expected outcomes related to quality of life

This type of outcome concerns general and specific dimensions that the profession defines as beneficial for people who receive care. These can include general health status, alleviation of signs or symptoms, acquisition of skill and knowledge, or improved abilities to function. Often the theory that is being used will suggest a specific outcome that is related to one or more general quality of life goals. These goals can guide the selection of the deliberative application outcome that you choose.

CONCLUSION

In this chapter we discussed how the activities of creating conceptual meaning and deliberative application of theory interact with practice to contribute to theory development. An individual nurse or group of nurses can select several options on how they might proceed with any of these activities, depending on the needs of their setting and clients. Having other individuals in the environment who understand and support these activities and who can give information and assistance is a tremendous asset.

Prerequisites to be considered before application of a theory in practice are discussed. Each of the prerequisites needs to be considered in order to make a sound judgment regarding application of theory. If the prerequisites are considered and application is made considering the guidelines offered here, nursing practice will indeed make a valuable contribution to theory development.

REFERENCES

Beckstrand JA: A critique of several conceptions of practice theory in nursing, Res Nurs Health 3(2):69-79, 1980.

Forsyth GL: Analysis of the concept of empathy: illustration of one approach, Adv Nurs Sci 2(2):33-42, 1980.

Schroeder PC and Maibusch RM, editors: Nursing quality assurance, Rockville, Md, 1984, Aspen.

Smeltzer C, Hinshaw A, and Feltman B: The benefits of staff nurse involvement in monitoring the quality of patient care, J Nurs Quality Assurance 1(3):1-7, 1987.

Appendix

INTERPRETIVE SUMMARY
Conceptual models in nursing:
1952-1981

The summaries provided here are not complete descriptions or critical reflections of the theorists' works. Rather, they are interpretive descriptions of the essential features of each conceptual model. They may be used as a basis for initial comparisons of theorists' works and as a basis for selecting a particular work for further description and critical reflection.

A notation of the definitive theoretic writing that each summary synthesizes precedes the summary. When theorists have multiple publications, the summaries focus on most recent ideas. The conceptual models are presented in the order shown in Table 3-6 (p. 52). The original terminology of the theorists has been retained.

H. E. Peplau
Interpersonal relations in nursing, 1952;
The art and science of nursing, 1988

The patient is an individual with a felt need, and nursing is a process that is both interpersonal and therapeutic. Nursing is the simultaneous application of art and science. The overall goal or purpose of nursing is to educate and be a maturing force so that personality development (a new view of self) occurs. This purpose is achieved when the nurse, as a medium for change, enters into a personal relationship with an individual, the patient, when a felt need presents itself. The personal relationship in nursing provides for meeting the individual patient's needs and assists two persons with different goals, that is, nurse and patient, to develop or assume congruent goals. The nurse-patient relationship occurs in phases during which the nurse functions as a resource person, a counselor, and a surrogate. The phases are four in number: orientation, identification, exploitation, and resolution. When a person with a need seeks help, the nurse assists in orientation to the problem. During phase one, the illness event is integrated. The person learns the facets of the difficulty and the extent of need for help. During phase one, orientation to use of services, productive exploitation of anxiety and tension, and learning the limits of necessary space and freedom occurs. This helps to ensure that the illness event is not repressed. When orientation is completed to a given degree, the phase of identification begins. In phase two the patient assumes a posture of interdependence, dependence, and/or independence in relation to the nurse. The nurse assists the patient during this phase, taking into consideration the services needed and the patient's history. Identification helps assure the patient that the nurse can understand the interpersonal meaning of the patient's situation. When identification is accomplished, phase three, exploitation, begins. In this phase the patient derives full value from the relationship by using the services available on the basis of self-interest and needs. Resolution, the final phase, occurs as old needs are met. With resolution of older needs, newer and more mature ones emerge. When needs are resolved, the person is freed from dependence on others. The maturing force of nursing is realized as the personality develops through the educational, therapeutic, interpersonal process of nursing. The phases of the relationship are serial and the patient assumes an active role.

During the dyadic nurse-patient relationship and greater nursing relationships with communities, many roles are assumed by nurses. These include roles of stranger, teacher, resource person, surrogate, leader, and counselor. Multiple roles occur as a result of multiple client problems and needs in individual interpersonal relationships, team functions, and variant social and professional expectations. The overall goal for professional nursing is the same as the nurse-patient dyads, that is, to implement a process that facilitates personality development by helping persons use forces and experiences to ensure maximum productivity.

F.G. Abdellah, I.L. Beland, A. Martin, and R.V. Matheney
Patient-centered approaches to nursing, 1960

The patient and/or family present with nursing problems that the nurse assists them to meet though her professional function. There are 21 problem categories that the nurse addresses. These relate to: (1) hygiene and physical comfort; (2) activity and rest; (3) safety; (4) body mechanics; (5) oxygenation; (6) nutrition; (7) elimination; (8) fluid and electrolytes; (9) responses to disease; (10) regulatory mechansims; (11) sensory function; (12) feelings and reactions; (13) emotions and illness interrelationships; (14) communication; (15) interpersonal relationships; (16) spirituality; (17) therapeutic environment; (18) awareness of self; (19) accepting limitations; (20) resources to resolve problems; and (21) role of social problems in illness.

Nursing problems are both overt or obvious and covert. Nurses must be aware of covert problems to meet care requirements. Overt and covert problems must be identified to make a nursing diagnosis. Identification of problems precedes solution. The nursing process is the method nurses use to establish and focus on a nursing diagnosis. The overall goal is fullest possible functioning for a client.

Individualized patient care is important for nursing. Both patients and nurses should be aware of the wholeness of clients, as well as the need for continuity of care from pre- to post-hospitalization. Individualized care will require changes in the organization and administration of nursing services, as well as educational changes.

I. J. Orlando
The dynamic nurse-patient relationship: function, process and principles, 1961; The discipline and teaching of nursing process: an evaluation study, 1972

The patient is an individual with a need, that is, a requirement that, if supplied, diminishes distress, increases adequacy, or enhances well-being. Needs include requirements for implementing physicians' plans, or other innate requirements. The nurse acts to meet needs and thus alleviate distress.

Patients with needs behave verbally and nonverbally in a given manner. The nurse reacts to patient behavior by ascertaining both the meaning of the distress and what would alleviate the distress. Finally, the nurse acts to alleviate distress noted. Distress can be due to (1) physical limitations, either temporary or permanent, (2) adverse reactions to the setting, such as being misinterpreted or misinterpreting, and (3) inability to communicate.

Three elements—patient behavior, nurse reactions, and nurse actions—comprise a nursing situation. Patient behavior and nurse reactions relate to the assessment phase of the nursing process and involve ongoing interaction with the nurse. Once the need is clearly ascertained through assessment, the nurse acts automatically or deliberatively. Automatic actions are those carried out for reasons other than resolving an immediate need, whereas deliberative actions seek to meet assessed needs. Automatic actions make problems by creating situational conflict that is evidenced through lack of resolution of needs and cooperation (i.e., distress is not alleviated).

Deliberative action yields solutions to problems and also prevents problems. Once the nursing action occurs, the nurse evaluates patient behavior to determine if the need has been met and resultant distress has been alleviated. The overall goal is to meet needs and, through that, to alleviate distress.

E. Wiedenbach
Clinical nursing: a helping art, 1964

The patient is an individual under treatment or care who experiences needs. Needs are requirements for maintenance or stability in a situation. Needs may be perceived by the individual as a requirement for help and may be met by the person or others. Also, persons may have needs and not seek help or may help themselves without recognizing a need. Needs for help are defined as measures or actions required and desired...which potentially restore or extend ability to cope with situational demands" (p. 6). Nursing is concerned with the needs that patients have for help. What the nurse does and how she or he does it comprise clinical nursing. Clinical nursing has four components: (1) philosophy, (2) purpose, (3) practice and art.

Philosophy is a personal stance of the nurse that embodies attitudes toward reality, and purpose is the overall goal. The purpose of clinical nursing is "to facilitate efforts of individuals to overcome obstacles which interfere with abilities to respond capably to demands made by the condition, environment, situation or time" (p. 15). The foregoing purpose is the embodiment of meeting needs for help. Meeting needs for help implies goal-directed, deliberate, patient-centered practice actions that require (1) knowledge (factual, speculative, and practical), (2) judgment, and (3) skills (procedural and communication). Practice includes four components: (1) identification of the perceived need for help, (2) ministration of help needed, (3) validation that help given was the help needed, and (4) coordination of help and resources for help—i.e., reporting, consulting, and conferring. The art of clinical nursing requires using individualized interpretations of behavior in meeting needs for help.

The helping process is triggered by patient behavior that is perceived and interpreted and in relation to which the nurse reacts. In interpreting behavior the nurse compares the perception to an expectation or hope. Nursing actions may be rational, reactionary, and deliberative. A rational response by the nurse is one based on the immediate perception without going beyond to explore hidden meaning. A reactionary response is one taken in reaction to strong feelings. Deliberative actions, the desirable mode, are those that intelligibly fulfill nursing's purpose. Identification of needs for help involves: (1) observing inconsistencies and acquiring information about how patients mean the cue given or determining the basis for an observed inconsistency, (2) determining the cause of the discomfort or need for help, and (3) determining whether the need for help can be met by the patient or whether assistance is required. Once needs for help are identified, ministration and validation that help was given follow.

The practice of clinical nursing is bounded by professional, local, legal, and personal constraints. Clinical nursing practice is supported by nursing administration, nursing education, nursing organizations, and nursing research. The clinical goal is to meet needs for help, integrating the practice and process of nursing. Greater professional goals include conservation of life and promotion of health.

L. E. Hall
Another view of nursing care and quality, 1966

The patient is a unity comprised of three overlapping parts: a person (the core aspect), a pathology and treatment (the cure aspect), and a body (the care aspect). The nurse is a bodily care giver. Provision of bodily care allows the nurse to comfort and to "gain entry" to the pathology and treatment aspect of the patient, as well as the person of the patient. Understanding, resulting from the integration of all three areas, allows the nurse to be an effective teacher and nurturer. The patient so managed learns and is nurtured in the person, that is, in the core aspect. Nurturance leads to effective rehabilitation: greater levels of self-actualization and self-love.

Nursing occurs during one of two phases of medical care. Phase one medical care is the diagnostic and treatment phase, and phase two is the evaluative, follow-up phase. The professional nurse's role is in phase two, and professional nursing practice requires a setting in which patients are free to learn. In phase two the nurse's goal is to help the patient learn. Motivation to learn is assured by advocating the patient's learning goals and not the doctor's curative goals. Once patient learning goals are codetermined with the nurse and motivation therefore assured, the patient will learn, and nurturance, rehabilitation, and self-love follow. The overall goal for the client is rehabilitation and consequently a greater measure of self-actualization and self-love.

V. Henderson
The nature of nursing, 1966

The patient is an individual who requires help toward independence. The nurse assists the individual, whether ill or not, to perform activities that will contribute to health, recovery, or peaceful death that the individual would perform unaided if he had necessary strength, will, or knowledge. The process of nursing strives to do this as rapidly as possible, and the goal is independence. The nurse manages this process independently of physicians. Help toward independence is given autonomously by the nurse in relation to (1) breathing, (2) eating and drinking, (3) elimination, (4) movement and posture, (5) sleep and rest, (6) clothing, (7) maintenance of body temperature, (8) cleaning and grooming of the body and integument protection, (9) avoiding environmental dangers and injury of others, (10) communication, (11) worship, (12) work, (13) play and participation in recreation, and (14) learning and discovery. Nursing can be evaluated as a profession based on the extent to which it achieves each of these functions autonomously.

The role and functions of professional nursing vary with the situation. If the total health care team comprises a "pie graph" in health care situations, there are some situations in which no role exists for certain health care workers. Although there is always a role for family and patients, "pie wedges" for team members vary in size according to (1) the problem of the patient, (2) the patient's self-help ability, and (3) help resources. Central to nursing that seeks to help patients toward independence is empathetic understanding and unlimited knowledge. Empathetic understanding grounded in genuine interest will lead to helping the family understand what a patient needs. The ultimate goal for the nurse is to practice autonomously in helping patients who lack knowledge, physical strength, or strength of will in growth toward independence. Because of this function, nurses will seek and promote research, education, and work settings that facilitate this goal.

J. Travelbee

Interpersonal aspects of nursing, 1966; Interpersonal aspects of nursing, 1971

Nursing is an interpersonal process aimed at assisting individuals, families, or communities to prevent or cope with the process of illness and suffering, and, if necessary, to find meaning in the experience. Nursing's purpose is achieved through human-to-human relationships, which are established by a disciplined intellectual approach to problems combined with therapeutic use of self. Human-to-human relationships require transcending roles of "nurse" and "patient" in order to establish relatedness and respond to the humanness of others. Nursing activities are a means to establishing relatedness and achieving nursing's purpose. The values and beliefs of nurses determine the quality of nursing care provided and thus the extent to which nurses are able to help the ill find meaning in their situation.

Illness and suffering are spiritual, emotional, and physical experiences. The nurse assists the ill patient to experience hope as a means of coping with illness and suffering. Communication, a central concept for Travelbee, implies guiding, planning, and purposely directing interaction to fulfill nursing's purpose. Communication is instrumental in establishing relatedness (knowing persons), ascertaining and meeting nursing needs, and in fulfilling nursing's purpose. Communication also implies that exchanged messages are understood. Communication techniques should enable the nurse to explore and understand the meaning of the person's communication. Establishment of the human-to-human relationship is phasic. The phases are: the original encounter, emerging identities, empathy, and sympathy (p. 119, ed. 2). In such a relationship the needs of the person are met. Achievement of a human-to-human relationship requires openness to experiences and freedom to use personal and experiential background to appreciate and understand the experiences of others.

Health and illness may be defined subjectively and objectively. Objective criteria are dependent on cultural and societal norms, whereas subjective criteria are peculiar to the human being. The meaning of the symptoms of illness (or criteria for health) for the person is more significant than affixing a label of health or illness to the effects or results of health or illness.

M. E. Levine

The four conservation principles of nursing, 1967; Introduction to clinical nursing, 1973; The conservation principles: twenty years later, 1989

Man is a holistic being whose open and fluid boundaries coexist with the environment. Environments may be perceptual, operational, and conceptual. Man is a unity who is to remain conserved and integral. He sends messages that reflect his current adaptive state. Adaptation is a method of change, and change is life process. When adaptation fails, conservation is threatened, and adaptation needs occur. Adaptive needs are reflected in messages sent.

Nursing occurs at the interface between the open and fluid boundaries of whole persons and environments. The nurse receives and interprets messages and intervenes supportively or therapeutically. Intervention is guided by the four principles of conservation: conservation of energy and structural, personal, and social integrity. Conservation, based on an assessment of man's adaptive needs, aids adaptation. When a patient's energy and structural, personal, and social integrity are conserved—that is, when the nurse acts therapeutically—adaptation can better occur, and man achieves a state of unity and integrity. When conservation cannot be effected in the face of overwhelming adaptation needs, death ensues. Supportive interventions are appropriate when adaptation is failing without hope of reversal, such as assisting a client toward peaceful death. The goal for nursing is the wholeness of the patient brought about by conservation in four areas when adaptive needs manifest.

M. E. Rogers
An introduction to the theoretical basis of nursing, 1970;
Nursing: a science of unitary man, 1980; Science of unitary human
beings: a paradigm for nursing, 1983; Nursing: a science of unitary
human beings, 1989

Man (unitary human being) is an energy field coextensive with the universe. Human-environment boundaries are only conceptually imposed and are arbitrary. The unity of human beings and environment is plausible, considering the sameness of matter and energy. Humans are more and different from the sum of their parts, and generalities about the whole cannot be made from a study of the parts. The energy comprising unitary human beings and environmental field is characterized by four dimensionality in which a given point in time is not tenable. The four concepts—energy fields, openness, pattern and organization, and four dimensionality—are used to derive principles that postulate how human beings develop. These principles are (1) integrality (formerly complimentarity), (2) resonancy, and (3) helicy. According to the principle of integrality, the human and environmental fields interact mutually and simultaneously. Resonancy postulates the nature of wave pattern changes as continuous from lower-frequency to higher-frequency patterns. Helicy asserts that field changes are innovative, probabilistic, and characterized by increasing diversity of field patterns.

Nursing seeks to care for unitary human beings in accordance with its science and art. Science is emergent and based on research and logical analysis of the principles of homeodynamics. Nursing science seeks to describe, explain, and predict. Art is the imaginative and creative use of knowledge and science. Nursing's goal is maximization of health potentials of individuals, family, and groups consistent with health's everchanging nature. Nursing then has as its goal to help people achieve well-being within the potential of family, group, and individual. This is achieved by artfully applying emerging science based on the principles of homeodynamics.

D. E. Orem
Nursing: concepts of practice, 1971; Nursing: concepts of practice, 1980;
Nursing: concepts of practice, 1985

Orem's self-care deficit theory of nursing includes theory of (1) self-care deficit, (2) self-care, and (3) nursing system. Self-care deficit theory postulates that people benefit from nursing in that they have health-related limitations in providing self-care. Self-care theory postulates that self-care and care of dependents are learned behaviors that purposely regulate human structural integrity, functioning, and development. Nursing systems theory postulates that nursing systems form when nurses prescribe, design, and provide nursing that regulates the individual's self-care capabilities and meets therapeutic self-care requirements.

Assumptions basic to the general theory are:
1. Humans require deliberate input to self and environment in order to be alive and to function.
2. The power to act deliberately is exercised in caring for self and others.
3. Mature humans will sometimes experience limitations in ability to care for self and others.
4. Humans discover, develop, and transmit ways to care for self and others.
5. Humans structure relationships and tasks to provide self-care.

Humans need continuous self-care maintenance and regulation and provide this by caring for self. Self-care enables purposeful action. Self-care activities maintain life, health, and well-being. Health refers to the state of a person, which is characterized by soundness or wholeness of developed human structures and bodily and mental functioning. Well-being refers to a person's perceived condition of existence, which is characterized by experiences of contentment, pleasure, happiness, movement toward self-ideals, and continuing personalization.

Three kinds of self-care requisites (requirements) are: universal, developmental, and health deviation. Universal requirements relate to the meeting of common human needs. Developmental self-care requisites relate to conditions that promote developmental processes throughout the life cycle. Health deviation self-care requisites relate to self-care that prevents defects and deviations from normal structure and integrity and those that control the extension and effects of such defects.

Adults care for themselves, whereas infants, the aged, the ill, and disabled persons require assistance with self-care activities. When self-care action is limited because of the health state or needs of the care recipient, nursing responds and provides a legitimate service. Thus patients are persons with health-related self-care deficits. Two variables affect these deficits: self-care agency (ability) and self-care demands.

Self-care agency is a learned ability and is deliberate action. Nurses, given their focus on care of patients with health-related limitations in self-care abilities, must accurately diagnose self-care agency. Thus they must have information about deficits and their reasons for existing. Such information is basic to selecting helping methods.

Nursing agency regulates or develops patient's self-care agency and ability to meet therapeutic self-care demand. Nursing is a helping service that involves acting or doing for another, guiding and supporting another, providing a developmental environment, and teaching another. Nursing agency varies with educational preparation; orientation to practice situations; mastery of technologies of practice; and ability to accept, work with, and care for others.

Nursing systems may be wholly compensatory, partially compensatory, or supportive-educative. Wholly compensatory systems are required for patients unable to control and monitor their environment and process information. Such patients are unable to control their movement and position and are unresponsive to stimuli. Partially compensatory systems are designed for patients with limitations in movement as a result of pathology or injury or who are under medical orders to restrict movements. Supportive-educative systems are designed for patients who need to learn to perform self-care measures and need assistance to do so. Nursing systems are formed to regulate self-care capabilities and meet therapeutic self-care requirements.

I. M. KING

Toward a theory for nursing: general concepts of human behavior 1971;
A theory for nursing: systems, concepts, process, 1981;
King's general systems framework and theory, 1989

The patient is a personal system within the environment who coexists with other personal systems. Individuals form groups that comprise interpersonal systems, and interpersonal systems contribute to social systems. Thus patient and nurse are comprised of personal systems as subsystems within interpersonal and social systems. The nurse must understand given aspects of all three systems. Concepts identified for each system affect total system function. There are three comprehensive concepts: perception for the personal system, organization for the social system, and interaction for the interpersonal system. Personal system concepts related to perception include self, body image, growth and development, time, space, and learning. The nurse also must have knowledge of role, communication, transaction, and stress to understand interactions central to interpersonal system function. Since interaction occurs within social systems, including family, belief, educational, and work systems, nurses require knowledge or organizational concepts of power, authority, control, status, and decision making in order to function adequately.

The focus for nursing is the human being in the system context. The goal is health. Health implies helping people in groups attain, maintain, and restore health, live with chronic illness or disability, or die with dignity. Interactions of the individual with the environment are significant in influencing life and health. Nurse and patient meet in a health care organization—patient needing help and nurse offering help. Nurse and patient perceive one another, act and react, interact and transact. In this process, presenting conditions are recognized, goal-related decisions are made, and motivation to exert control over events to achieve goals occurs. Transactions are basic to goal attainment and include social exchange, bargaining and negotiating, and sharing a frame of reference toward mutual goal setting. Transactions require perceptual accuracy in nurse-client interactions and congruence between role performance and role expectation for nurse and client. Transactions lead to goal attainment, satisfaction, effective care, and enhanced growth and development. The goal of nursing process interaction is transaction, which leads to attainment of goals set in relation to health promotion, maintenance, and recovery from illness.

B. Neuman
The Betty Neuman health-care systems model: a total person approach to patient problems, 1974; The Neuman systems model, 1982; The Neuman systems model, 1989

The person is a unique, holistic system, yet possesses a common range of normal characteristics and responses. Persons are a dynamic composite of physiologic, psychologic, sociocultural, developmental, and spiritual variables. These variables interact with internal and external environmental stressors. The holistic system of the person is open. As an open system it interacts with, adjusts to, and is adjusted by the environment. The external environment is (defined as) all that interfaces with the person's system. The internal and external environments are a source of stressors that have different potentials to disturb the normal line of defense. Stressors, which penetrate the normal line of defense, disrupt the system. The normal line of defense is essentially the usual steady state of the individual and is comprised of the normal range of responses to stressors within persons which evolve over time. The flexible line of defense cushions and protects individuals from stressors. Lines of resistance are conceptualized as internal factors that help persons defend against stressors. Lines of resistance protect the core structure and stabilize and return individuals to a normal line of defense when stressors break through.

The system's model is based on an individual's relationship to stress, the reaction to it, and reconstitution factors that are dynamic in nature. The nurse assesses, manages, and evaluates patient systems. Nursing's focus is the variables that affect a person's response to stressors. Assessment of individuals considers knowledge of factors influencing a patient's perceptual field, the meaning stressors have to patient as validated by patient and caregiver, and factors the caregiver believes influence the patient situation. Basically, nursing focuses on the occurrence of stressors, the organism's response to them, and the state of the organism. Primary prevention identifies and allays risk factors associated with stressors; it focuses on protecting the normal line of defense and strengthening the flexible line of defense. Secondary prevention is related to symptomatology, intervention priorities, and treatment; it helps to strengthen internal lines of defense. Death occurs if the basic core structure of the system fails to support the intervention. Tertiary prevention protects reconstitution or return to wellness following treatment.

Nursing acts to impede or to arrest an entropic state, or a state of disorder and disorganization. Health is a state of movement toward negentropy or evolution; it is a state of inertness free from disrupting needs. Health implies a homeostatic balance. This balance depends on free energy flow between the organism and the environment. In health the system's normal line of defense is maintained, and the lines of resistance are intact; the basic structural elements of the system are preserved.

Appendix

Sister C. Roy

Introduction to nursing: an adaptation model, 1976; The Roy adaptation model, 1980; Theory construction in nursing: an adaptation model, 1981; Introduction to nursing: an adaptation model, 1984; The Roy adaptation model, 1989

The person is an adaptive system. System inputs include (1) three classes of stimuli (focal, contextual, or residual) that arise from within the person and the external environment and (2) adaptation level. Adaptation level is fluid, is comprised of all three classes of stimuli, and respresents the person's standard or range of stimuli in which responses will be adaptive.

Inputs are mediated by the control process subsystems of cognator and regulator coping mechanisms. The regulator mechanism is an automatic neuroendocrine response, whereas the cognator subsystems represent perception, information processing, and judgments influenced by learning and emotions. Coping activity may or may not be adequate to maintain integrity. A system difficulty presents when coping actvity is inadequate as a result of need excesses or deficits.

The system effectors are the adaptive modes. These modes (physiologic, self-concept, role function, and interdependence) are the form in which regulator and cognator subsystems manifest their activity.

The adaptive system (person's) output is a response that may be adaptive or ineffective. Adaptive responses are those that contribute to adaptation goals—i.e., responses that promote growth, survival, reproduction, and self-mastery. Adaptation is an ongoing purposive response. Adaptive responses contribute to health, the process of being and becoming integrated; ineffective responses do not.

Using nursing process, the nurse promotes adaptive responses in the adaptive modes during health and illness. Thus energy is freed from inadequate coping to promote health and wellness. System responses in each mode are assessed—i.e., described using objective and subjective data (first-level assessment). Behaviors can be assessed by observation, measurement, and interviewing. A tentative judgment about whether the behavior is adaptive or ineffective is then made. Stimuli influencing the adaptive system are then identified (second level assessment). A nursing diagnosis follows, goals are set, and interventions selected. Goals are mutually agreed upon, and a goal-setting heierarchy proposed. Survival is a priority goal, followed by goals that promote growth, ensure continuation of the race or society, and promote attainment of full potential. Factors precipitating ineffective behavior are changed, and coping behavior (i.e., adaptation level) is broadened. The person's level of coping is continuously revised. Evaluation of interventions requires returning to the first steps in the nursing process—i.e., noting behaviors manifest by the adaptive system or person.

J. G. Paterson and L. T. Zderad
Humanistic nursing, 1976

Man is a unique being, extant in all nursing situations, who innately struggles "to know." Humanistic nursing is an existential experience of being and doing with such that nurturance in relation—in the between—with another occurs. Fundamentally, nursing is a response to human need and can be described to build a humanistic nursing science.

Humanistic nursing requires that the participants be aware of their uniqueness, as well as their commonality with others. Authenticity is required—an in-touchness with self that comes in part with experiencing. Humanistic nursing also presupposes responsible choices. The ability of an individual to make choices based on authentic awareness and knowledge of such choices are concerns of humanistic nursing and cultivate moreness. Also, a commitment to the value of humanistic nursing must be present.

A nurse with the foregoing attitudes and qualities can offer genuine presence to another. Humanistic nursing concerns the basic nursing act: the response of one human in need to another. At this level, nursing is related to the health-illness quality of the human condition: nurturance toward more being.

M. M. Leininger
Transcultural nursing: concepts, theories, and practices, 1978; Caring: a central focus of nursing and health care services, 1980; The phenomenon of caring: importance, research questions and theoretical considerations, 1981; Leininger's theory of nursing: cultural care diversity and universality, 1988

Caring is postulated as the central and unifying domain for nursing knowledge and practices. Diverse factors influence patterns of care and health or well-being in different cultures. Caring includes assistive, supportive, and facilitative acts toward or for another individual or a group with evident or anticipated needs. Caring serves to ameliorate or to improve human conditions or life ways. Professional caring includes behaviors, techniques, processes, and patterns that improve or maintain healthy conditions or lifeways. Professional nursing care embodies scientific and humanistic modes of helping or enabling receipt of personalized service to maintain a healthy condition for life or death.

Caring emphasizes healthful, enabling activities of individuals and groups that are based on culturally defined ascribed or sanctioned helping modes. Caring behaviors include the following: comfort, compassion, concern, coping behavior, empathy, enabling, facilitating, interest, involvement, health consultative acts, health instruction acts, health maintenance acts, helping behaviors, love, nurturance, presence, protective behaviors, restorative behaviors, sharing, stimulating behaviors, stress alleviation, succorance, support, surveillance, tenderness, touching, and trust (1981, p. 13). Culture determines personal life or world views that are mediated through language. Contextual factors such as technology, religion, philosophic beliefs, social and kinship lines and patterns, values and life ways, political and legal factors, economic, and educational factors all influence care patterns. Likewise these factors affect care patterns and health of individuals, families as well as groups. Diverse health systems mediate the expression of health. Nursing is one health system that overlaps with folk systems and professional health care systems.

Human caring is a universal phenomenon, and every nursing situation has transcultural nursing care elements. Caring is essential to human development, growth, and survival, and caring behaviors vary transculturally in priorities, expression, and needs satisfaction. Caring plays a more important role in recovery than cure but receives less reward. If effective, caring reflects professional concern, compassion, stress alleviation, nurturance, comfort, and protection. Nursing is to provide care consistent with its emergent science and knowledge, with caring as a central focus. Caring and culture are inextricably linked, and nursing care should be culturally congruent and aimed at preserving, maintaining, accommodating, negotiating, repatterning, and restructuring care patterns.

J. Watson
Nursing: the philosophy and science of caring, 1979; Nursing: human science and human care, 1985; New dimensions of human caring theory, 1988; Watson's philsosophy and theory of human caring in nursing, 1989

Assumptions underlying human care values in nursing include: (1) care and love comprise the primal and universal psychic energy, and (2) care and love are requisite for our survival and the nourishment of humanity. Caring for and loving self is requisite to caring for others. Curing is not the end to be sought but is a means to care. Nursing's ability to sustain its caring ideology and translate it into practice will determine its contribution to society. Nursing has traditionally held a caring stance in relation to patients with health and illness concerns, and caring is the unifying focus for practice in nursing. Caring has received little emphasis in the health care system, and caring values of nursing are critical to sustaining care ideals in practice. Preservation of human care is a significant issue; human care can be practiced only interpersonally; and nursing's social, moral, and scientific contributions lie in its commitment to human care ideals. The foregoing assumptions provide a rationale for developing nursing as a human science.

Humans are capable of transcending time and space and possess a spirit, soul, or essence that enables self-awareness, higher degrees of consciousness, and a power to transcend the usual self. Human life is a continuous (with time and space) being in the world. Caring, an intersubjective human process, is the moral ideal of nursing. Human care processes have an energy field and involve engagement of mind-body-soul with another in a lived moment. Illness, not necessarily disease, is a state of subjective turmoil in which self as "I" is separated from self as "me." Conversely, health is a harmony within mind-body-soul in which the "I" and "me" are aligned. A healthy person is open to increased diversity. The goal of nursing is to help persons increase harmony within mind-body-soul, which leads to self knowledge, self reverence, self-healing, and self care.

Theoretic premises identified include the following. At nursing's highest level the nurse makes contact with the person's emotional and subjective world as the route to inner self; mind and soul are not confined in time and space and to the physical universe; a nurse can access inner self through the mind-body-soul, provided the physical body is not perceived separate from the higher sense of self. The geist (spirit or inner self) exists in and for itself and relates to the human ability to be free—love and caring are universal givens; illness may be hidden from the "eyes" and require the finding of meaning in inner experiences. Finally, the totality of experiences at the moment constitute a phenomenal field or the individual's frame of reference.

Persons strive to satisfy needs experienced in the perceived phenomenal field. These include being cared for, loved, and valued and experiencing positive regard, acceptance, and understanding. Persons also strive to achieve union, transcend individual life, and find harmony with life. All needs are subservient to a basic striving toward actualizing spiritual self and establishing harmony within mind-body-soul. Harmony is consistent with a sense of congruence between "I" and "me" self as perceived, and self as experienced, as well as congruence between subjective reality (phenomenal field) and external reality (world as is).

Caring occasions involve action and choice by nurse and individual. If the caring occasion is transpersonal, the limits of openness are expanded as are human capacities. Transpersonal caring relationships depend on moral commitments to enhance human dignity to allow persons to determine their own meaning, the nurse's affirmation of the subjective significance of the person, the nurse's ability to detect feelings of another's inner condition and feel a union with another, and the nurse's history of living and experiencing feelings and human conditions and imagining others' feelings; that is, personal growth, maturation, and development of the nurse's self.

Nursing interventions related to human care are referred to as carative factors and include nurturing, forming, cultivating, and using: (1) humanistic-altruistic system of values, (2) faith-hope, (3) sensitivity to self and others, (4) helping-trusting human care relationship, (5) expressing positive and negative feelings, (6) creative problem solving caring process, (7) transpersonal teaching-learning, (8) supportive, protective, and/or corrective mental, physical, societal, and spiritual environment, (9) human needs assistance, and (10) existential-phenomenological spiritual forces. Carative factors are actualized in the human care process.

M. A. Newman
Theory development in nursing, 1979; Newman's health theory, 1983;
Health as expanding consciousness, 1986

Individuals are subsumed by a greater whole and are part of multiple system levels in space. Explicit assumptions are made in relation to health, pathology, and patterns. Health can encompass pathology and disease; therefore, disease and health are not continuous variables or opposites. Pathology manifests according to a preexisting unitary pattern. Thus disease gives clues to the pattern of a person's life, and pattern is reflected in energy exchange within humans and between humans and environment. Personal patterns manifesting as disease are part of larger patterns, which are not altered when the disease is eliminated. Disease as a pattern manifestation may be considered health. The existence of disease may evoke tension, an important evolutionary ingredient. Disease is not advocated as a desirable state, but the significance of attending to the meaning of the disease is highlighted. Health is an expansion of consciousness, and pattern-manifesting disease expands consciousness.

Consciousness, the informational capacity of the system, is reflected in both the quality and quantity of responses to stimuli. Health involves developing awareness of self and environment coupled with increased ability to perceive and respond to alternatives. Movement is a central concept, a property of life. The concepts of consciousness, time, movement, and space are interrelated in that movement reflects consciousness and is an identifiable and specific individual characteristic. Time is an index of consciousness and a function of movement. Movement is the means whereby time and space become reality, and space and time have a complimentary relationship. Without movement, time and space are not real, and there is no change at any system level. Movement reflects the organization of consciousness and therefore reflects health. The implied goal is consciousness expansion and therefore health and life. Health is not a state but an experienced process.

D. E. JOHNSON
The behavioral system model for nursing, 1980

The individual patient is a behavioral system comprised of subsystems. As a behavioral system, the patient's subsystems strive to maintain balance, making adjustments to factors impinging on them. Humans seek experiences that may disturb balance and require behavior modifications to reestablish balance. Behavioral systems are essential and reflect adaptations that are successful. The behavioral system is comprised of behaviors that form an integrated unit. Behavioral systems maintain their own integrity, link individuals with environment, and are self-perpetuating if environmental conditions remain orderly and predictable. The multiple tasks of behavioral systems require continual system changes, including subsystem evolution. Subsystems also must be protected, nurtured, and stimulated.

Behavioral system subsystems are formed from responses or response tendencies that share a common goal and are modified by maturation and experience. Each subsystem of the overall behavioral system has a specialized task or function that can be described on the basis of that structure and function. There are four structural elements in each subsystem: (1) drive-stimulated or goal sought, (2) set or predisposition to act in a given way, (3) choices, or scope of action alternatives, and (4) behavior. Only the last structural element is observable. Seven subsystems are identified: (1) attachment or affiliative, (2) dependency, (3) ingestive, (4) eliminative, (5) sexual, (6) aggressive, and (7) achievement. The attachment subsystem responses provide security, and dependency provides for nurturance responses. The ingestive and eliminative subsystems relate to eating and excretion of waste. The sexual subsystem relates to the dual responses of procreation and sexual fulfillment. The aggressive subsystem functions to preserve the person, and the achievement system functions so that mastery of self and the environment is fostered.

Nursing problems manifest when subsystems cannot maintain a dynamic stability or when the subsystem has not achieved an optimum level of function. Anticipated problems in subsystems can be prevented, and manifest problems solved. The nurse acts to impose a regulatory mechanism, change structural units, and fulfil functional requirements of subsystems. The nursing act seeks to "preserve the organization and integration of the patient's behavior at an optimal level under those conditions in which the behavior constitutes a threat to physical or social health, or in which illness is found" (p. 214).

R. R. PARSE
Man-living-health: a theory of nursing, 1981; man-living-health:
a man-environment simultaneity paradigm, 1985;
A nursing science: major paradigms, theories, critiques, 1987;
A man-living-health: a theory of nursing, 1989

Man is unitary, that is, an indivisible being who interrelates with the environment while cocreating health. Theoretic assumptions synthesize the concepts of energy field, openness, pattern and organization, four dimensionality, helicy, integrality, coconstitution, coexistence, and situated freedom with tenets of human subjectivity and intentionality. Assumptions (nine in the 1981 work have been reduced to three in the 1987 work) state that man is a recognizable pattern who evolves simultaneously with environment. Man-environment relationships are such that a continuity of what was and what will be unfolds in the now. Man chooses the meaning given to cocreated situations and is responsible for choices made. Unitary man is recognized by individual patterns of relating, which are cocreated in man-environment interchange. There is mutual man-environment interrelatedness as man chooses to move toward irreversible possibilities. Man experiences in multiple dimensions simultaneously and relatively. The negentropic interchange of man-environment both enables and limits becoming.

Health is an open process of becoming, an incarnation of man's choosings. As man-environment connect and separate, health is cocreated. Thus health is a synthesis of values cocreated in open interchange with environment. Health is a continuous process of transcending with the possibles, that is, reaching beyond the actual. Health is an emergent: a negentropic unfolding.

The theory of man-living-health emerges from the stated assumptions, and three principles are notable:

> "structuring meaning multidensionally is cocreating reality through the languaging of valuing, and imaging; (2) cocreating rhythmical patterns of relating is living the paradoxical unity of revealing-concealing and enabling-limiting while connecting-separating; (3) cotranscending with the possibles is powering unique ways or originating in the process of transforming" (1987, p. 163).

Principle one asserts that reality is continually cocreated by assigning meaning to all-at-once experiences occurring multidimensionally. Imaging, valuing, and languaging serve to structure meaning multidimensionally. Principle two asserts that there is an unfolding cadence of coconstituting ways of being. Ways of being are recognized in the man-environment interchange and are lived rhythmically. Rhythms of revealing-concealing, enabling-limiting, and connecting-separating are integral in the principles. The final principle asserts that concepts of cotranscending with the possibles—powering, originating, and transforming—are mans' ways of aspiring toward the "not-yet. Three theoretic structures are posited:

> "(1) powering is a way of revealing and concealing imaging; (2) originating is a manifestation of enabling and limiting valuing; and (3) transforming unfolds in the languaging of connecting and separating" (1981, p. 68).

REFERENCES

Abdellah FG et al: Patient-centered approaches to nursing, New York, 1960, The Macmillan Co.

Hall LE: Another view of nursing care and quality. In Straub KM and Parker KS, editors: Continuity pf patient care: the role of nursing, Washington, DC, 1966, Catholic University Press, pp 47-60.

Henderson V: The nature of nursing, New York, 1966, The Macmillan Co.

Johnson DE: The behavioral system model for nursing. In Riehl JP and Roy Sr C: Conceptual models for nursing practice, ed 2, New York, 1980, Appleton-Century-Crofts, pp 207-216.

King IM: Toward a theory for nursing: general concepts of human behavior, New York, 1971, John Wiley & Sons.

King IM: A theory for nursing: system, concepts, process, New York, 1981, John Wiley & Sons.

King IM: King's general systems framework and theory. In Riehl-Sisca J, editor: conceptual models for nursing practice, ed 3, Norwalk, Conn, 1989, Appleton & Lange, pp 149-158.

Leininger MM: Transcultural nursing: concepts, theories, and practices, New York, 1978, John Wiley & Sons.

Leininger MM: Caring: a central focus of nursing and health care services, Nurs Health Care 1(3): 135-143, 1980.

Leininger MM: The phenomenon of caring: importance, research questions and theoretical considerations. In Caring: an essential human need (Proceedings of the three national caring conferences), Thorofare, NJ, 1981, Charles B Slack, Inc, pp 3-15.

Leininger MM: Leininger's theory of nursing; cultural care diversity and universality, Nurs Sci Q 1(4):152-160, 1988.

Levine ME: The four conservation principles of nursing, Nurs Forum, 6(1):45-59, 1967.

Levine ME: Introduction to clinical nursing, Philadelphia, 1973, FA Davis Co.

Levine ME: The conservation principles: twenty years later. In Riehl-Sisca J, editor, Conceptual models for nursing practice, ed 3, Norwalk, Conn, 1989, Appleton & Lange, pp 325-337

Neuman B: The Betty Neuman health care systems model: a total person approach to patient problems. In Riehl JP and Roy Sr C, editors: Conceptual models for nursing practice, ed 2, New York, 1980, Appleton-Century-Crofts, pp 119-131.

Neuman B: The Neuman systems model, Norwalk, Conn, 1982, Appleton-Century-Crofts.

Neuman B: The Neuman systems model, ed 2, Norwalk, Conn, 1989, Appleton & Lange.

Newman MA: Theory development in nursing, Philadelphia, 1979, FA Davis Co.

Newman MA: Newman's health theory. In Clements IW and Roberts FB, editors: Family health: a theoretical approach to nursing care, New York, 1983, John Wiley & Sons, pp 161-175.

Newman MA: Health as expanding consciousness, St. Louis, 1986, Mosby–Year Book, Inc.

Orem DE: Nursing: concepts of practice, New York, 1971, McGraw-Hill Book Co, Inc.

Orem DE: Nursing: concepts of practice, ed 2, New York, 1980, McGraw-Hill Book Co, Inc.

Orem DE: Nursing: concepts of practice, ed 3, New York, 1985, McGraw-Hill Book Co, Inc.

Orlando IJ: The dynamic nurse-patient relationship: function, process, and principles, New York, 1961, G.P. Putman's Sons.

Orlando IJ: The discipline and teaching of nursing process: an evaluation study, New York, 1972, G.P. Putman's Sons.

Parse RR: Man-living-health: theory of nursing, New York, 1981, John Wiley & Sons.

Parse RR: Nursing science: major paradigms, theories and critiques, Philadelphia, 1987, WB Saunders.

Parse RR: Man-living-health: a theory of nursing. In Riehl-Sisca J, editor: Conceptual models for nursing practice, ed 3, Norwalk, Conn, 1989, Appleton & Lange, pp 253-257.

Parse RR, Coyne AB, and Smith MJ: Nursing research: Qualitative methods, Bowie, Md, 1985, Brady Communications Co, pp 9-13.

Paterson JG and Zderad LT: Humanistic nursing, New York, 1976, John Wiley & Sons.

Peplau HE: Interpersonal relations in nursing, New York, 1952, GP Putnam's Sons.

Peplau HE: The art and science of nursing: similarities, differences, and relations, Nurs Sci Q 9(1):8-15, 1988.

Rogers ME: An introduction to the theoretical basis of nursing, Philadelphia, 1970, FA Davis Co.

Rogers ME: Nursing: a science of unitary man. In Riehl JP and Roy Sr C, editors: Conceptual models for nursing practice, ed 2, New York, 1980, Appleton-Century-Crofts, pp 329-337.

Rogers ME: Science of unitary human beings: a paradigm for nursing. In Clements IW and Roberts FB, editors: Family health: a theoretical approach to nursing care, New York, 1983, John Wiley & Sons, pp. 219-228.

Rogers ME: Nursing: a science of unitary human beings. In Riehl-Sisca J, editor: Conceptual models for nursing practice, ed 3, Norwalk, Conn, 1989, Appleton & Lange, pp 181-188.

Roy Sr C: Introduction to nursing: an adaptation model, Englewood Cliffs, 1976, Prentice-Hall, Inc.

Roy Sr C: The Roy adaptation model. In Riehl JP and Roy Sr C, editors: Conceptual models for nursing practice, ed 2, New York, 1980, Appleton-Century-Crofts, pp 179-188.

Roy, Sr. C: Introduction to nursing: an adaptation model, ed 2, Norwalk, Conn, 1984, Appleton-Century-Crofts.

Roy Sr C: The Roy adaptation model. In Riehl-Sisca J, editor: Conceptual models for nursing practice, ed 3, Norwalk, Conn, 1989, Appleton & Lange, pp 105-114.

Roy Sr C and Roberts S: Theory construction in nursing: an adaptation model, Englewood Cliffs, 1981, Prentice-Hall, Inc.

Travelbee, J: Interpersonal aspects of nursing, Philadelphia, 1966, FA Davis Co.

Travelbee, J: Interpersonal aspects of nursing, ed 2, Philadelphia, 1971, FA Davis Co.

Watson J: Nursing: the philosophy and science of caring, Boston, 1979, Little, Brown & Co.

Watson J: Nursing: human science and human care, Norwalk, Conn, 1985, Appleton-Century-Crofts.

Watson J: New dimensions of human caring theory, Nurs Sc Q 9(4):175-181, 1988.

Watson J: Watson's philosophy and theory of human caring, In Riehl-Sisca J, editor: Conceptual models for nursing practice, ed 3, Norwalk, Conn, 1989, Appleton & Lange, pp 219-236.

Wiedenbach E: Clinical nursing: a helping art, New York, 1964, Springer Publishing Co, Inc.

Glossary

This glossary provides definitions for words with multiple meanings, as well as those used with a particular meaning in this text. Undefined words are used consistent with standard dictionary definitions. The page numbers following each entry indicate where additional information about the word may be located.

abstract concept Mental image derived from more indirect evidence that is not easily represented by a specific empiric indicator. The meaning of abstract concepts contained in theories can be derived from the context of the theory and often do not have the same meaning in common language. Because abstract concepts are constructed from indirect evidence, they are often interpreted differently by different people and are influenced by an individual's own perceptions and experience. (p. 58)

accessibility Trait of theory that refers to the degree to which concepts have indicators in observable reality. (p. 135)

armchair theory Common language term that refers to a theory constructed from mental images without the use of research methods. Armchair theory may be developed using logic and rational argument. Armchair theory may also imply the causal compilation of ideas without reference to systematic processes. (p. 63)

art/act Form in which esthetic knowing in nursing is expressed. Each art/act is unique and particular and cannot be replicated. (p. 10)

assumption Something that is taken for granted or thought to be true without systematically generated empiric evidence. Theoretic assumptions may be taken as "truth" because they cannot be empirically tested, as in a value statement. Assumptions may have potential for empiric testing, but are taken to be true because they are consistent with a world view or are judged to be reasonable. Assumptions may also have a degree of empiric confirmation but are designated as assumptions within theory because they do not comprise the major focus of theoretic reasoning. The term "assumption" may be used synonymously with "supposition," as when something is taken as "truth for the sake of argument." (pp. 96, 118)

atomistic theory Theory that deals with a narrow scope of phenomena. The term often implies, in addition, an assumption that the whole may be understood from a study of the parts. This term may be used synonymously with the terms "micro" and "molecular" theory. (p. 123)

axiom Type of premise used in deductive logic, often one that is not tentative, but relatively firm. Axioms as premises are used for deducing theorems, especially in mathematics. (p. 65)

choice The fundamental purpose toward which all knowing is directed; the outcome of integration of empiric, esthetic, ethical, and personal knowledge. (pp. 6, 48)

clarity Trait that refers to the lucidity and consistency of the theory. (pp. 129, 132)

components of theory Features of theory that are useful for discribing theory. Components include purpose, concepts, definitions, relationships, structure, and assumptions. (p. 108)

concept Complex mental formulation of empiric experience. Concepts are a major component of theory and convey the abstract ideas within the theory. (pp. 58, 80)

conceptual framework/model Structure comprised of concepts related to form a whole. Descriptive theoretic statements may be called conceptual models or frameworks. (pp. 39, 75)

conclusions Relationship statements that are derived from premises in a deductive logic system. Conclusions are a type of proposition and may take the form of a theorem or hypothesis. (p. 64)

consensus Process for forming understanding that emerges from the esthetic pattern of knowing. This process requires bringing to conscious awareness the diverse perspectives of others and integrating and integrating knowledge of those perspectives. Consensus and criticism interact to provide a means for understanding the meaning of esthetic knowledge. (p. 13)

consistency Trait related to clarity. Consistency may be semantic or structural and refers to the general agreement, harmony, and compatibility of components within the theory. (pp. 131, 133)

construct Type of highly abstract and complex concept whose reality base can only be inferred. Constructs are formed from multiple less abstract or more empiric concepts. (p. 60)

creating conceptual meaning Theory development process of identifying, examining, and clarifying the mental images that comprise the elements, variables, or concepts within theory. (pp. 27, 80, 163)

creative dimension of knowing Process of knowing that draws on experience and moves toward what might be in the future. (p. 5)

criteria for concepts Essential features of a concept formed by examining conceptual meaning. Criteria are designed with reference to the purposes for which the concept is being used and should be useful to both identify and differentiate the concept from other concepts. (p. 90)

criteria for nursing diagnoses Essential features for a specific diagnosis to be used in a given instance or situation encountered in nursing practice. (p. 166)

critical reflection Process that addresses questions concerning the function, purposes, and value of empiric theory. (p. 128)

criticism Process for forming understanding that emerges from the esthetic pattern of knowing. Criticism is deliberate, critical, precise, and thoughtful reflection and action directed toward transformation. Consensus and criticism interact to provide a means for understanding the meaning of esthetic knowledge. (p. 13)

deduction Form of reasoning that moves from the general to the specific. In *deductive logic,* two or more premises as relational statements are used to draw a conclusion. In *deductive research processes,* an abstract theoretic relationship is used to derive specific questions or hypotheses. (p. 64)

definition Component of theory that indicates the empiric basis for a concept. Definitions are statements of meaning that provide a link between theoretic abstractions and empiric indicators. Definitions may be relatively general or specific. Theoretic definitions refer to the conceptual meaning of a term, whereas operational definitions specify how the concept is empirically assessed. (pp. 61, 94, 112)

deliberative application of theory Theory development process for testing the usefulness of theory in practice. This process draws on research methods and places theory within the context of nursing practice to ensure that theory serves the goals of the profession. (pp. 28, 102, 167)

descriptive relationships Statements that provide an account of what something is. Descriptive relationships provide a specific image or impression of the nature or attributes of a phenomenon. (p. 113)

dialogue Process for forming understanding that arises from ethical knowing in nursing. Dialogue is an exchange of various points of view concerning what is "right," "good," "responsible." This process, in interaction with the process of justification, provides a means for challenging, rethinking, reforming, and clarifying ethical knowledge. (p. 13)

direct observation Perception of the existence of an object, property, or event by sensory means. Perception occurs at the time the phenomenon exists in reality in such a way that the object, property, or event can be objectively verified as present by more than one observer. (pp. 58, 163)

discipline Group of individuals engaged in developing a body of knowledge, the structured knowledge within an area of concern or domain of inquiry. (pp. 2, 46)

empiric-abstract continuum Means to visualize or represent the extent to which concepts have a basis in empiric reality. Empiric concepts have a direct reality basis, whereas abstract concepts have an indirect basis in empiric reality. (p. 58)

empiric concept Mental image derived from relatively direct sensory experience. A concept that represents an object, property, or event is referred to as empiric when it is experienced by the senses and can be verified and similarly described by many different observers. Empiric concepts are often more easily represented by empiric indicators than abstract concepts and can be directly observed. (p. 58)

empiric indicators Object, property, or event that is verifiable in reality; the sensory experience related to a concept. Concrete concepts have more direct empiric indicators; abstract concepts require the construction of indirect measures or tools that provide an approximate empiric measurement of some feature of the phenomenon. (pp. 58, 100, 135, 153, 163)

empiric testing Systematic means of validating empiric reality or of observing and assessing phenomena that occur in reality. Empiric testing usually implies that research methods are used in the process of validation. (pp. 28, 99)

empiric theory Theory that expresses empiric knowledge in nursing, drawing on ideas about human science and nursing as a practice professsion. (p. 20)

empirics The pattern of knowing in nursing that is the science of nursing, expressed in scientific-empiric theories. (pp. 7-8)

esthetics The pattern of knowing in nursing based on comprehension of meaning, expressed in an art/act. (pp. 10-11)

ethical principles or guidelines Statements that express the values upon which nursing actions are based. (p. 9)

ethical theory Type of theory that is developed to justify value positions. The concepts of ethical theory may be operationalized empirically, but empiric reality is not adequate for judging the validity of the theory. The adequacy of the theory is judged by the consistency of logic against the underlying value assumptions on which the theory is based. (p. 9)

ethics Pattern of knowing in nursing focusing on moral knowledge, expressed as principles and guidelines. (p. 8)

explanatory relationships Statements that provide ideas about how events happen, indicating how related factors affect or result in certain phenomena. (p. 113)

expressive dimensions of knowing Ways in which nursing's patterns of knowing are communicated and shared. Empirics and ethics are expressed in verbal forms: personal knowing and esthetics are expressed in human actions and behavior. (p. 5)

fact Objectively verifiable event, object, or property; a phenomenon that is reported similarly by more than one person. (p. 75)

general definition A statement of the meaning of a term or concept that sets forth characteristics of the phenomenon or what the phenomenon is associated with. A specific definition, by contrast, states particular characteristics, or indicators, that name what the phenomenon is. (p. 112)

generality Trait of theory that refers to the range of phenomena to which the theory applies. Generality combined with simplicity yields parsimony. (p. 134)

generalizability Extent to which research findings can be applied to or used as a basis for making decisions in like situations. Generalizability is affected by the soundness of the conceptualization process, the research design, and the analysis of the data. (p. 158)

generating and testing theoretic relationships Theory development process that includes (1) empirically grounding emerging relationships, (2) explicating empiric indicators, and (3) validating the relationships through empiric methods. (pp. 28, 99)

grand theory Theory that deals with broad goals and concepts representing the total range of phenomena of concern within a discipline. This term may be used to imply "macro," "molar," and "holistic" theory. (p. 123)

grounded theory Theory generated from inductive research processes; the source of data is empiric reality. (pp. 147, 155)

holism (wholism) Perspective that is based on the assumption that a whole cannot be reduced to discrete elements or be analyzed without residue into the sum of its parts. Holism may also refer to an emphasis or value of the whole but with consideration of discrete parts that are interrelated. (p. 46)

holistic theory Theory that deals with a broad scope of phenomena. A theory of high-level wellness is holistic in comparison to a theory of pain alleviation. Use of the term "holistic theory" often implies, in addition, an assumption that the "whole" is greater than the sum of its parts. This term may be used to imply "macro" and "grand" theory. (p. 123)

hypothesis Tentative statement of relationship between two or more variables that can be empirically tested. The term "hypothesis" is generally used to refer to a relationship statement that is tested using specific research methods. (pp. 63, 149)

Glossary

importance Trait of theory that refers to the extent to which a theory is clinically significant or has value for the profession. (p. 136)

indirect observation Perception of phenomenon or methods that assess properties or traits from which the existence of the phenomenon can be inferred. (pp. 58, 153)

induction Form of reasoning that moves from the specific to the general. In inductive *logic*, a series of particulars are combined into a larger whole or set of things. In inductive *research*, particular events are observed and analyzed as a basis for formulating general theoretic statements, often called "grounded" theory. (p. 65)

integration Process required for and arising from determining the credibility of all patterns of knowing. (p. 14)

isolated research Research that is completed without recognized reference or linkage to theory. (p. 142)

justification Process for forming understanding that arises from ethical knowing in nursing; justification provides an explicit description of the values on which an ethical idea rests and the line of reasoning toward which an ethical conclusion flows. This process, in interaction with the process of dialogue, provides a means for clarifying, reforming, rethinking, and challenging ethical knowledge. (p. 13)

knowing Individual human processes of experiencing and comprehending self and the world in ways that can be brought to some level of conscious awareness. Not all that is comprehended in the processes of knowing can be shared or communicated. That which is shared, communicated, and expressed in words or in actions becomes knowledge. (p. 5)

knowledge Awareness or perception of reality acquired through insight, learning, or investigation expressed in a form that can be shared. (p. 5)

law Relationship between variables that has been thoroughly tested and confirmed. Laws are said to be highly generalizable and are relatively certain. (p. 65)

logic System of reasoning that deals with the form of relationships among propositions without specific regard to their content. (p. 64)

macro theory Theory that deals with a broad scope of phenomena. This term may be used to imply "grand," "molar," and "holistic" theory. (p. 124)

meta theory Theory about the nature of theory and the processes for its development. (p. 123)

micro theory Theory that is relatively narrow in scope or deals with a narrow range of phenomena. This term may be used to imply "atomistic" and "molecular" theory. (p. 123)

midrange theory Theory that deals with a relatively broad scope of phenomena but does not cover the full range of phenomena that are of concern within a discipline. A theory of pain alleviation represents a midrange theory for nursing; it is broader than a theory of neural conduction of pain stimuli but narrower than the goal of achieving high-level wellness. The phenomenon of pain is a midrange concept of concern for nursing because it is only one of many phenomena that comprise the global concern of the discipline. (pp. 53, 124)

model General term referring to symbolic representation of perceptual phenomena. Models may provide a sense of understanding as to how theoretic relationships develop and are useful to illustrate various forms of theoretic relationships. Models may also be physical objects that replicate certain features of the larger object, as in a model train. (p. 75)

molar theory Theory that deals with a broad scope of phenomena. This term may be used to imply "grand," "macro," and "holistic" theory. (p. 123)

molecular theory Theory that is relatively narrow in scope of deals with a narrow range of phenomena. This term may be used to imply "micro" and "atomistic" theory. (p. 123)

nursing practice Experiences a nurse encounters in the process of caring for people. Experiences include those of the person receiving care, the nurse, others in the environment, and their interactions. (pp. 21, 109)

objectivity Assumption upon which methods of science are based, in which truth is thought to exist apart from or outside of the person who knows. Based on a dualistic view of the rational mind and "out there" reality as separate. (p. 3)

operational definition Statement of meaning that indicates how a term or concept can be assesed empirically. Operational definitions are inferred from theoretic definitions. They specify the empiric indicator(s) selected for the purpose of developing research and the means of observing and measuring the indicator(s). (p. 65)

paradigm Generally accepted structure or world view within a discipline that organizes the processes and outcomes of inquiry, including theory. (p. 76)

parsimony Relative trait of theory that incorporates degrees of both simplicity and generality. A highly parsimonious theory is one that has a broad range or generality, yet is stated in very simple terms. (p. 134)

patterns gone wild The distortion that occurs when any one pattern of knowing is not critically examined and integrated with the whole of knowing. (p. 15)

personal knowing Pattern of knowing in nursing focused on inner experience and becoming a whole, aware self. (p. 9)

philosophy Form of disciplined inquiry for the purpose of discerning general traits of reality. (p. 75)

predictive relationships Set of statements that interrelates variables such that a specified outcome can be expected when the theory is used. (pp. 98, 114)

premises Relationship statements that are used in deductive logic as a basis for forming a conclusion. In logic, the form of the argument must be valid, regardless of how sound the premises are. Examples of types of premises include hypotheses and axioms. (p. 64)

principle Brief statement of value and/or fundamental truth that is to be followed in providing nursing care. It may also refer to principles of practice, often derived from accepted facts or theoretic propositions from other disciplines. (p. 36)

processes for forming understanding Process that provides a means for integrating the significance, background, meanings, facts, and experiences that form the whole of knowing. These processes include critical questions that are addressed and sociopolitical processes of interaction that arise from the distinct nature of each pattern of knowing in nursing. Once the processes of forming understanding are engaged, the processes make all patterns accessible and create movement between and among the processes for the other patterns of knowing. (p. 11)

processes for theory development In a practice discipline, the processes for theory development are: creating conceptual meaning, structuring and contextualizing theory, generating and testing theoretic relationships, and deliberative application of theory. (p. 27)

profession Vocation that requires specialized knowledge, provides a role in society that is valued, and uses some means of internal regulations of its members. (p. 47)

proposition Statement of relationship between two or more variables. The term "proposition" is a general category that includes "postulates," "premise," suppositions," "axioms," "conclusions," "theorems," and "hypotheses." When a distinction in meaning is made between these various terms, the distinction reflects the form or purpose of logic used or the context in which the proposition occurs. For example, a hypothesis is generally used in the context of a research study. "Axiom" and "theorem" are used to refer to the relationship statements that are made in a particular type of deductive logic. (p. 63)

purpose Reasons underlying a theory's development; the outcome or outcomes expected to emerge if the relationships of the theory are valid. The purpose of the theory also suggests the range of situations in which the theory is expected to apply. (p. 108)

reductionism Philosophic stance that the whole can be partitioned and understood through generalizations made from a study of the parts. (p. 42)

reflection Process for forming understanding that arises from personal knowing in nursing. Reflection is an inner process that requires integrating a wide range of perceptions in order to actually realize what is known within the self of the knower. Reflection interacts with response to form a process of growth in understanding the self as genuine and authentic. (p. 13)

relationship statements Any statement that sets forth a connection or association between two or more phenomena. This general term is used to denote both tentative and confirmed types of statements, such as propositions, laws, axioms, and hypotheses. As a more general term, it does not imply a particular form of logic or a particular context in which the statement is used. (p. 98)

relationships Component of theory that refers to the interconnections between concepts. (p. 113)

replication Process for forming understanding that arises from empiric knowing in nursing. This process draws on methods of science to determine the extent to which an observation remains consistent from one situation or time to another. This process interacts with the process of validation to form clear and accurate understanding of empiric knowledge. (p. 13)

research Application of systematic methods of empirics in order to develop knowledge. (pp. 75, 142)

response Process for forming understanding that arises from personal knowing in nursing. Response is what arises from others who experience the self; it reflects or "mirrors back" the self of the knower. Reflection interacts with response to foster growth in understanding the self as genuine and authentic. (p. 13)

science Body of knowledge, including facts and theories generated by the use of rigorous and precise methods within an area of concern; the process of using rigorous and precise methods to generate facts and theories within an area of concern. Natural science assumes invariant laws of nature that are separate from the scientist. Human science assumes that the scientist constructs, in part, what is known. (p. 74)

Glossary

simplicity Trait of theory that refers to the degree to which a theory reduces complexity by using a minimum number of descriptive components, especially concepts, to accomplish its purpose. Simplicity implies that the theory has the fewest number of conceptual ideas in relationship that are required. Simplicity combined with generality yields parsimony. (p. 133)

social/political process Interactive methods that are designed for each of the patterns of knowing and that contribute to the integrating process of forming understanding. The methods require an individual and group interaction within the dynamic cultural, political and social context of the times. The interactive processes are: empirics—replication/validation, ethics—dialogue/justification, personal knowing—response/reflection, and esthetics—consensus/criticism. (p. 12)

specific definition Statement of the meaning of a term or concept that names the associated object, property, or event and assigns particular characteristics to the object, property, or event as opposed to saying what the concept is like or associated with in reality. (p. 112)

structure Trait of theory that refers to the morphologic arrangement of relationships within the theory. (p. 114)

structuring and contextualizing theory Theory development process of organizing relationships between and among concepts in a rigorous and systematic way, consistent with the purposes of the theory. This process also includes the processes of identifying the domain, realm, or context of the theory; stating the assumptions upon which the theory is based; and providing conceptual definitions of terms that guide decisions about the empiric events to which concepts relate. (pp. 28, 93)

theorem Conclusion that is drawn from axioms as premises in a deductive form of logic. Theorems and axioms are used most often in logical sciences such as mathematics, and the relationships expressed imply some degree of certainty or validity. (p. 65)

theoretic definition Statement of meaning that conveys essential features of a concept in a manner that fits meaningfully within the theory. A theoretic definition specifies conceptual meaning and implies empiric indicators for concepts. This word may be used synonymously with conceptual definition. (p. 96)

theoretic framework/model Structure comprised of concepts related in some way to form a whole. The term "theoretic framework" or "model" often connotes less tentativeness than conceptual framework or model, but often theoretic and conceptual model and framework are used interchangeably. (p. 75)

theory Creative and rigorous structuring of ideas that project a tentative, purposeful, and systematic view of phenomena. (p. 71)

theory-linked research Research that is designed with reference or linkage to theory. Theory-linked research may be theory testing or theory generating. Theory-testing research ascertains how accurately existing theoretic relationships depict reality-based events. Theory-generating research is designed to discover and describe relationships by observing empiric reality and then constructing theory based on empiric data observed. (p. 142)

validation Process for forming understanding that arises from empiric knowing in nursing. Validation is a process that focuses on the accuracy of conceptual meanings in terms of empiric evidence. Validation and replication interact to provide a means of forming clear and accurate understandings of empiric knowledge. (p. 13)

Bibliography

Abdellah FG: The nature of nursing science, Nurs Res 18(5):390-393, 1969.

Abdellah FG et al: Patient centered approaches to nursing, New York, 1960, The Macmillan Co.

Allen D: Nursing research and social control: alternative models of science that emphasize understanding and emancipation, Image, J Nurs Scholarship 17(2):59-64, 1985.

Allan JD and Hall BA: Challenging the focus on technology: a critique of the medical model in a changing health care system, Adv Nurs Sci 10(3):22-34, 1988.

Ashley JA: Foundations for scholarship: historical research in nursing, Nurs Sci (1):25-36, 1978.

Barzun J and Graff HF: The modern researcher, ed 4, New York, 1985, Harcourt Brace.

Beckstand J: A critique of several conceptions of practice theory in nursing, Res Nurs Health 3(2):69-79, 1980.

Benner P: From novice to expert: excellence and power in clinical nursing practice, Menlo Park, 1984, Addison-Wesley.

Benner P: Quality of life: a phenomenological perspective on explanation, prediction, and understanding in nursing science, Adv Nurs Sci 8(1):1-14, 1985.

Benner P and Wrubel J: The primacy of caring, Menlo Park, 1989, Addison-Wesley.

Benoliel JA: The interaction between theory and research, Nurs Outlook 25(2):108-113, 1977.

Berthold JS: Theoretical and empirical clarification of concepts, Nurs Sci 2(5):406-422, 1964.

Berthold JS: Symposium on theory development in nursing: prologue, Nurs Res 17(3):196-197, 1968.

Bleicher J: Contemporary hermeneutics: hermeneutics as method, philosophy and critique, Boston, 1980, Routledge and Keegan Paul.

Bok S: Lying: moral choice in public and private life, New York, 1978, Pantheon Books.

Boulding KE: The image, Ann Arbor, 1961, University of Michigan Press.

Butterfield PG: Thinking upstream: nurturing a conceptual understanding of the societal context of health behavior, Adv Nurs Sci 12(2):1-8, 1990.

Carper BA: Fundamental patterns of knowing in nursing, Adv Nurs Sci 1(1):13-23, 1978.

Carper BA: The ethics of caring, Adv Nurs Sci 1(3):11-19, 1979.

Chinn PL, editor: Advances in nursing theory development, Rockville, Md, 1983, Aspen Systems Corp.

Chinn PL: Debunking myths in nursing theory and research, Image, J Nurs Scholarship 17(2):45-49, 1985.

Chinn PL: The art of criticism, editorial, Adv Nurs Sci 7(4):vii-viii, 1985.

Chinn PL: Nursing research methodology, Rockville, Md, 1986, Aspen Systems Corp.

Chinn PL: Nursing patterns of knowing and feminist thought, Nurs Health Care, 19(2):71-75, 1989.

Chinn PL and Jacobs MK: A model for theory development in nursing, Adv Nurs Sci 1(1):1-11, 1978.

Chinn PL and Wheeler CE: Feminism and nursing, Nurs Outlook, 33(2):74-77, 1985.

Clements IW and Roberts FB: Family health: a theoretical approach to nursing care, New York, 1983, John Wiley & Sons.

Curtin LL: The nurse as advocate: a philosophical foundation for nursing, Adv Nurs Sci 1(3):1-10, 1979.

Davenport NJ: The nurse scientist—between two worlds, Nurs Outlook 28(1):28-31, 1980.

DeGroot HA: Scientific inquiry in nursing: a model for a new age, Adv Nurs Sci 10(3):1-21, 1988.

Dickoff J and James P: A theory of theories: a position paper, Nurs Res 17(3):197-203, 1968.

Dickoff J and James P: Clarity to what end? Nurs Res 20(6):499-502, 1971.

Dickoff J and James P: Organization and expansion of knowledge: toward a constructive assault on the imperious distinction of pure from applied knowledge, of knowledge from technology, Dent Hyg 62(1):15-20, 1988.

Dickoff J, James P, and Wiedenbach E: Theory in a practice discipline. Part I: Practice-oreinted theory, Nurs Res 17(5):415-435, 1968.

Donaldson SK and Crowley DM: The discipline of nursing, Nurs Outlook, 26(2):113-120, 1968.

Downs FS: Nature of relationship between theory and practice. In Ketefian S, editor: Translation of theory into nursing practice and education: proceedings of the seventh annual clinical sessions, New York, 1975, New York University Division of Nursing, pp 1-9.

Ellis R: Characteristics of significant theories, Nurs Res 17(3):217-222, 1968.

Ellis R: The practitioner as theorist, Am J Nurs 69(7):1434-1438, 1969.

Ellis R: Commentary on Walker's "Toward a clearer understanding of the concept of nursing theory," Nurs Res 20(6):493-494, 1971.

Fawcett J: The relationship between theory and research: a double helix, Adv Nurs 1(1):49-62, 1978.

Fawcett J and Downs FS: The relationship of theory and research, Norwalk, Conn, 1986, Appleton-Century-Crofts.

Fawcett J: Analysis and evaluation of conceptual models of nursing, ed 2, Norwalk, Conn, 1989, Appleton & Lange.

Feinstein AR: Clinical judgment, Hudington, NY, 1967, Robert E. Kreiger Publishing Co, Inc.

Fitzpatrick J and Whall A, editor: Conceptual models of nursing: analysis and application, ed 2, Norwalk, Conn, Appleton & Lange, 1989.

Flaskerud JH and Halloran EJ: Areas of agreement in nursing theory development, Adv Nurs Sci 3(1):1-7, 1980.

Fry ST: Toward a theory of nursing ethics, Adv Nurs Sci 11(2):9-22, 1989.

Fulton JS: Virginia Henderson: theorist, prophet, poet, 10(1):1-9, 1987.

George J, editor: Nursing theories: the basis for professional practice, ed 3, Norwalk, Conn, 1990, Appleton & Lange.

Gilligan C: In a different voice: psychological theory and women's development, Cambridge, 1982, Harvard University Press.

Giorgi A: Psychology as a human science: a phenomenologically based approach, New York, 1970, Harper & Row Publishers, Inc.

Glaser B and Strauss A: The discovery of grounded theory, Chicago, 1967, Aldine Publishing Co.

Gortner SR: The history and philosophy of nursing science and research, Adv Nurs Sci 5(2):1-8, 1983.

Greene JA: Science, nursing and nursing science: a conceptual analysis, Adv Nurs Sci 2(1):57-64, 1979.

Griffin AP: Philosophy and nursing, J Adv Nurs 5(3):261-272, 1980.

Hagan KL: Internal affairs: a journalkeeping workbook for self-intimacy, New York, 1990, Harper & Row.

Hall LE: A center of nursing, Nurs Outlook, 11(11):805-806, 1963.

Hall LE: Another view of nursing care and quality. In Straub KM and Parker KS, editors: Continuity of patient care: the role of nursing, Washington DC, 1966, Catholic University Press, pp 47-60.

Hardy ME, editor: Theoretical foundations for nursing, New York, 1973, MSS Information Corp.

Henderson V: The nature of nursing, New York, 1966, The Macmillan Co.

Hinshaw AS: Theoretical substruction: an assessment process, West J Nurs Res 1(4):319-324, 1979.

Howard RJ: The three faces of hermeneutics, Berkeley, 1980, University of California Press.

Jacobs MK: Can nursing theory be tested? In Chinn PL, editor: Methodological issues in nursing, Rockville, Md, 1986, Aspen Publishers.

Bibliography

Jacobs-Kramer MD and Chinn PL: Perspectives on knowing; a model of nursing knowledge, Scholarly Inquiry Nurs Pract 2(2):129-139, 1988.

Jacobs MK and Huether SE: Nursing science: the theory-practice linkage, Adv Nurs Sci 1(1):63-73, 1978.

Jacox A: Theory construction in nursing: an overview, Nurs Res 23(1):4-13, 1974.

Jennings BM and Meleis AI: Nursing theory and administrative practice: agenda for the 1990s, Adv Nurs Sci 10(3):56-69, 1988.

Johnson DE: Theory in nursing: borrowed and unique, Nurs Res 17(3):206-209, 1968.

Johnson DE: The behavioral system model for nursing. In Riehl JP and Roy Sr C, editors: Conceptual models for nursing practice, ed 2, New York, 1980, Appleton-Century-Crofts, pp 207-216.

Johnson, DE: "Some thoughts on nursing," Clin Nurs Spec 1(2):1-4, 1989.

Kaplan A: The conduct of inquiry, New York, 1964, Thomas Y. Crowell Co, Inc.

King IM: A theory of nursing: systems, concepts, process, New York, 1981, John Wiley & Sons.

King IM: King's general systems framework and theory. In Riehl-Sisca J, editor: Conceptual models for nursing practice, ed 3, Norwalk, Conn, 1989, Appleton & Lange, pp 149-158.

Kramer MK: Holistic nursing: implications for knowledge development and utilization. In Chaska NL, editor: The nursing profession: turning points, St. Louis, 1990, Mosby-n-Year Book, Inc, pp 245-254.

Krieger D: Foundations for holistic health nursing practices: the renaissance nurse, Philadelphia, 1981, JB Lippincott Co.

Krueter FR: What good is nursing care? Nurs Outlook 5(5):302-304, 1957.

Kuhn T: The structure of scientific revolution, Chicago, 1972, The University of Chicago Press.

Laudan L: Progress and its problems, Berkeley, 1977, University of California Press.

Leddy S and Pepper JM: Conceptual bases of professional nursing, ed 2, Philadelphia, 1989, JB Lippincott Co.

Leininger MM: Transcultural nursing: concepts theories and practices, New York, 1978, John Wiley & Sons.

Leininger MM: Care: the essence of nursing and health, Thorofare, NJ, 1984, Charles B Slack, Inc.

Leininger MM: Leininger's theory of nursing; cultural care diversity and universality, Nurs Sci Q 1(4):152-160, 1988.

Leonard VW: A Heideggerian phenomenologic perspective on the concept of the person, Adv Nurs Sci 11(4):40-55, 1989.

Levine ME: The four conservation principles of nursing, Nurs Forum 6(1):45-59, 1967.

Levine ME: Introduction to clinical nursing, ed 2, Philadelphia, 1973, FA Davis Co.

Levine ME: The conservation principles: twenty years later. In Riehl-Sisca J, editor: Conceptual models for nursing practice, ed 3, Norwalk, Conn, 1989, Appleton & Lange, pp 325-337.

MacPherson KI: Feminist methods: a new paradigm for nursing research, Adv Nurs Sci 5(2):17-26, 1983.

Malinski VM: Explorations on Martha Rogers: science of unitary human beings, Norwalk, Conn, 1986, Appleton-Century-Crofts.

Marriner-Tomey, A, editor: Nursing theorists and their work, ed 2, St. Louis, 1989, Mosby-n-Year Book, Inc.

McKay RP: Theories, models and systems for nursing, Nurs Res 18(5):393-399, 1969.

Meleis A: Theoretical nursing, Philadelphia, 1985, JB Lippincott Co.

Melosh B: The physician's hand: work culture and conflict in American nursing, Philadelphia, 1982, Temple University Press.

Merton RK: The sociology of science: theoretical and empirical investigations, Chicago, 1973, The University of Chicago Press.

Moccia P: A critique of compromise: beyond the methods debate, Adv Nurs Sci 10(4):1-9, 1988.

Moccia P: A further investigation of "dialectical thinking as a means of understanding systems-in-development: relevance to Roger's principles," Adv Nurs Sci 7(4):33-38, 1985.

Moccia P, ed: New approaches to theory development, New York, 1986, National League for Nursing.

Munhall PL: Nursing philosophy and nursing research: in apposition or opposition? Nurs Res 31(3):176-177, 1982.

Bibliography

Munhall PL: Methodological fallacies: a critical self-appraisal, Adv Nurs Sci 5(4):41-50, 1983.

Munhall PL: Methodological issues in nursing research: beyond a wax apple, Adv Nurs Sci 8(3):1-5, 1989.

Murphy JF: Theoretical issues in professional nursing, New York, 1971, Appleton-Century-Crofts.

Neuman B: The Neuman systems model, ed 2, Norwalk, Conn, 1989, Appleton & Lange.

Newman MA: Health as expanding consciousness, St. Louis, 1986, Mosby–Year Book, Inc.

Nicoll LH, ed: Perspectives on nursing theory, Boston, 1986, Little, Brown & Co.

Nightingale F: Notes on nursing: what it is and what is it not, New York, 1969, Dover Publications. (Unabridged republication of the first American edition, as published in 1860 by D. Appleton & Co.)

Noddings N: Caring: A feminine approach to ethics and moral education, Berkeley and Los Angeles, 1984, University of California Press.

Norris CM, editor: Proceedings of the first, second and third nursing conferences, Kansas City, Ks, 1969-1970, University of Kansas Medical Center Department of Nursing Education.

Norris CM: Concept clarification in nursing, Rockville, Md, 1982, Aspen Systems Corp.

Nursing theory: a circle of knowledge, Parts I and II, Video Tape, New York, National League for Nursing.

Omery A: Phenomenology: a method for nursing research, Adv Nurs Sci 5(2):49-64, 1983.

Orem D: Nursing: concepts of practice, ed 3, New York, 1985, McGraw-Hill Book Co, Inc.

Orlando IJ: The dynamic nurse-patient relationship: function, process, and principles, New York, 1961, G.P. Putnam's Sons.

Orlando IJ: The discipline and teaching of nursing process: an evaluation study, New York, 1972, G.P. Putnam's Sons.

Parse RR: Nursing science: major paradigms, theories and critiques, Philadelphia, 1987, WB Saunders.

Parse RR: Man-living-health: a theory of nursing. In Riehl-Sisca J, editor: Conceptual models for nursing practice, ed 3, Norwalk, Conn, 1988, Appleton & Lange, pp 253-257.

Paterson JG: From a philosophy of clinical nursing to a method of nursology, Nurs Res 29(2):143-146, 1971.(Republished by the National League for Nursing, 1987.)

Peplau HE: Interpersonal relations in nursing, New York, 1952, G.P. Putnam's Sons.

Peplau HE: The art and science of nursing: similarities, differences, and relations, Nurs Sci Q 1(1):8-15, 1988.

Polkinghorne D: Methodology for the human sciences, Albany, 1983, SUNY Press.

Popper KR: Conjectures and refutations: the growth of scientific knowledge, New York, 1965, Basic Books.

Quint JC: The case for theories generated from empirical data, Nurs Res 16(2):109-114, 1967.

Ramos MC: Adopting an evolutionary lens: an optimistic approach to discovering strength in nursing, Adv Nurs Sci 10(1):19-26, 1983.

Reed PG: Nursing theorizing as an ethical endeavor, Adv Nurs Sci 11(3):1-10, 1989.

Reichenbach H: The rise of scientific philosophy, Berkeley, 1951, University of California Press.

Reverby SM: Ordered to care: the dilemma of American nursing, 1850-1945, New York, 1987, Cambridge University Press.

Reynolds PD: A primer in theory construction, Indianapolis, 1971, The Bobbs-Merrill Co, Inc.

Riehl-Siosca, JP, editor: Conceptual models for nursing practice, ed 3, Norwalk, Conn, 1988, Appleton & Lange.

Roberts H, editor: Doing feminist research, Boston, 1981, Routledge and Kegan Paul.

Roberts SJ: Oppressed group behavior: implications for nursing, Adv Nurs Sci 5(4):21-30, 1983.

Rogers ME: An introduction to the theoretical basis of nursing, Philadelphia, 1970, FA Davis Co.

Rogers ME: Nursing: a science of unitary human beings. In Riehl-Sisca J, editor: Conceptual models for nursing practice, ed 3, Norwalk, Conn, 1988, Appleton & Lange.

Roy Sr C: Introduction to nursing: an adaptation model, ed 2, Norwalk, Conn, 1984, Appleton-Century-Crofts.

Roy Sr C: The Roy adaptation model. In Riehl-Sisca J, editor: Conceptual models for nursing practice, ed 3, Norwalk, Conn, 1989, Appleton & Lange, pp 105-114.

Roy Sr C and Roberts S: Theory construction in nursing: an adaptation model, Englewook Cliffs, 1981, Prentice-Hall, Inc.

Sandelowski M: The problem of rigor in qualitative research, Adv Nurs Sci 8(3):27-37, 1986.

Sarter B: Evolutionary idealism: a philosophical foundation for holistic nursing theory, Adv Nurs Sci 9(2)1-9, 1987.

Sarter B, editor: Paths to knowledge: Innovative research methods for nursing, New York, 1989, National League for Nursing.

Schlotfeldt RM: Nursing research: reflection of values, Nurs Res 26(1):4-9, 1977.

Schlotfeldt RM: Nursing in the future, Nurs Outlook 29(5):295-301, 1981.

Schultz PR and Meleis AI: "Nursing epistemology: traditions, insights, questions," Image, J Nurs Scholarship 20(4):217-224, 1988.

Silva MC: Research testing nursing theory: state of the art, Adv Nurs Sci 9(1):1-11, 1986.

Smith JA: The idea of health: implications for the nursing professional, New York, 1983, Teachers College Press.

Spender D: Manmade language, Boston, 1980, Routledge and Kegan Paul.

Stern PN: Grounded theory methodology: its uses and processes, Image, J Nurs Scholarship 12(1):20-23, 1980.

Stevens BJ: Nursing theories: one or many? In Grace HK and McCloskey JC, editors: Current issues in nursing, Boston, 1981, Blackwell Scientific Publications, pp 35-43.

Stevens BJ: Nursing theory: analysis, application and evaluation, ed 2, Boston, 1984, Little, Brown & Co.

Stevens BJ: Nursing theory: analysis and evaluation, ed 3, Glenview, Ill, 1990, Scott Foresman, Little, Brown & Co.

Stevens PE: A critical social reconceptualization of environment in nursing: implications for methodology, Adv Nurs Sci 11(4):56-68, 1989.

Theories at work, Video Tape, New York, National League for Nursing.

Theory development: What? Why? How? New York, 1978, National League for Nursing.

Thibodeux JA: Nursing models: analysis and evaluation, Monterey, 1983, Wadsworth Health Sciences Division.

Thompson JL: Practical discourse in nursing: going beyond empiricism and historicism, Adv Nurs Sci 7(4):59-71, 1985.

Thompson JL: Critical scholarship: The critique of domination in nursing, Adv Nurs Sci 19(1):27-38, 1987.

Tong R: Feminist thought: a comprehensive introduction, Boulder and San Francisco, 1989, Westview Press.

Travelbee J: Interpersonal aspects of nursing, Philadelphia, 1966, FA Davis Co.

Travelbee J: Interpersonal aspects of nursing, ed 2, Philadelphia, 1971, FA Davis Co.

Twomey JG, Jr: Analysis of the claim to distinct nursing ethics: normative and non-normative approaches, Adv Nurs Sci 11(3):25-32, 1989.

Walker LO and Avant KC: Strategies for theory construction in nursing, ed 2, Norwalk, Conn, 1988, Appleton & Lange.

Watson J: New dimensions of human caring theory, Nurs Sci Q, 1(4):175-181, 1988.

Watson J: Nursing: the philosophy and science of caring, Boston, 1979, Little, Brown & Co.

Watson J: Nursing: human science and human care, Norwalk, Conn, 1985, Appleton-Century-Crofts.

Watson J: Watson's philosophy and theory of human caring. In Riehl-Sisca J, editor: Conceptual models for nursing practice, ed 3, Norwalk, Conn, 1988, Appleton & Lange, pp 219-236.

Wheeler CE and Chinn PL: Peace and power: a handbook of feminist process, ed 2, New York, 1989, National League for Nursing.

Wiedenbach E: Clinical nursing: a helping art, New York, 1964, Springer Publishing Co, Inc.

Williams DM: Political theory and individualistic health promotion, Adv Nurs Sci 12(1):14-25, 1989.

Bibliography

Wilson J: Thinking with concepts, London, 1963, Cambridge University Press.

Winstead-Fry P, editor: Case studies in nursing theory, New York, 1986, National League for Nursing.

Winstead-Fry P: The scientific method and its impact on holistic health, Adv Nurs Sci 2(4):1-7, 1980.

Yeo M: Integration of nursing theory and nursing ethics, Adv Nurs Sci 11(3):33-42, 1989.

Index

A

A priori knowing, 3
Abdellah's summary of conceptual model, 177
Abstract concept, 196
  empiric concept and, 58–60
  nursing theory complexity and, 58–62
Abstraction, systematic, 20–21
Accessibility, 196
  of theory, 135–136
Adaptation model of nursing, 187
Advocating in ethics, 9
Ambiguity, 62
Armchair theory, 196
Art/act, 11, 196
Assumption, 196
  in theory, 96–97, 108, 118–119
Atomistic theory, 196
Authority, 3
Axiom, 196

B

Barrier, theory as, 144
Behavioral system model for nursing, 192–193
Beland's theory of nursing, 177
Benner's theory of person, 44
Benner and Wrubel's phenomenologic/hermeneutic method of inquiry, 48
Body
  of knowledge, 2
  mind versus, 4
Borderline cases as data source, 87–88
Boundary lines, theory development and, 30
Broad to specific structural idea form, 116

C

Cardiovascular fitness as concept, 59
Care, perceived quality of, 172
Caring
  phenomenon of, 188–189
  philosophy and science of, 189–191
  theory of human, 189–191
Carper's patterns of knowing, 4
Cases as data source, 85–87
Causation, conceptual meaning and, 95
Centering in personal knowing, 10
Choice, 197
Clarifying in ethics, 9
Clarity, 197
  critical reflection and, 129–133
  semantic, 130–131
  structural, 132–133
Classification of theory, 124
Clinical setting, theory usefulness for, 103, 169–170; see also Practice
Coherence of purpose, 23–24
Communication
  pain management and, 25
  professional, 25–26
Complex to simple structural idea form, 116
Concept, 57–77
  abstract, 196
    empiric concept and, 58–60
    nursing theory complexity and, 58–62
  abstract complexity and, 58–62
  comparative analysis of definitions and, 62–71
  comprehensive definition and, 71–73
  criteria for, 90–92, 197
  definition of, 58–59, 61–62, 197
    cup example in, 61–62
  definition of terms and, 74–76
  differentiation of similar, 164–165
  empiric, 198; see also Empirics
    abstract concept and, 58–60
  formation of, 81
  identification of new, 165–166
  intervening, 95
  of practice, 183–184

Concept—cont'd
  selection of, 83
  of theory, 108, 111–113
  in theory development, 94–96
  understanding of, 61–62
Conceptual, 69
Conceptual framework, 197
  Dickoff and James' definition of, 70
Conceptual meaning, 197
  approach to, 82
  clarification of purpose and, 84
  data sources and, 84–89
  exploration of contexts and values and,
      89–90
  formulating criteria for, 90–92
  problems and, 92–93
  selection of concept and, 83
  in theory development, 27, 80–93
Conceptual model, 175–195, 197
  of Abdellah, Beland, Martin, and
      Matheney, 177
  chronology of, 52
  early; see Early nursing models
  of Hall, 179–180
  of Henderson, 180
  in history of nursing theory, 39–40
  interpretive summary of, 175–195
  of Johnson, 192–193
  of King, 184–185
  of Leininger, 188–189
  of Levine, 181–182
  of Neuman, 185–186
  of Newman, 191–192
  of nursing; see Nursing conceptual model
  of Orem, 183–184
  of Orlando, 177–178
  of Parse, 193–194
  of Paterson and Zderad, 188
  of Peplau, 176–177
  of Rogers, 182–183
  of Roy, 187
  of Travelbee, 181
  of Watson, 189–191
  of Wiedenbach, 178–179
Conclusion, 197
  in theory-linked research, 156–158
Congruence, goal, 168–169
Consciousness, health as expanding, 191–
      192
Consensus, 197
  understanding and, 13–14
Conservation principles of nursing, 181–182

Consistency, 197
  semantic, 131–132
  structural, 133
Construct, 60, 197
Context
  clarification of, 97
  in determining theory usefulness, 169
  theory development and, 89–90, 97
  of theory emergence, 48–51
Contextualizing of theory, 28, 203
  assumptions and, 96–97
  clarifying context in, 97
  concepts and, 94–96
  designing relationship statements in, 98–
      99
Continuum, structural idea form of, 116,
      117
Contrary cases as data source, 86–87
Creating of conceptual meaning; see
      Conceptual meaning
Creative dimension of knowing, 7, 197
Criteria
  for concepts, 90–92, 197
  for empathy, 165
  for nursing diagnosis, 166–167, 197
Critical reflection, 127–139, 197
  accessibility and, 135–136
  clarity and, 129–133
  generality and, 134–135
  guide for, 138–139
  importance and, 136–137
  reasons for, 128–129
  simplicity and, 133–134
Criticism, 197
  understanding and, 13–14
Cultural care diversity and universality, 188–
      189

D

Data
  sources of, 84–89
    cases as, 85–88
    definitions as, 84–85
    literature as, 88, 89
    music as, 88–89
    people as, 89
  theory-linked research
    analysis of, 156–158
    obtaining of, 153–154
Deduction, 197
  in research processes, 197

Index

Deductive logic, 64–65, 197
  versus induction, 67–68
Definition, 198
  ambiguity in, 62
  of concept, 58–59, 61–62, 197
  as data source in conceptual meaning, 84–85
  general, 199
  operational, 201
  specific, 203
  theoretic, 203
  of theory; *see* Theory, definition of
Deliberative application of theory, 102–104, 198
Description
  in empirics, 8
  of theory, 107–126; *see also* Theory, description of
Descriptive relationships, 198
Development
  of research, 149–158; *see also* Research, development of
  of theory, 79–105; *see also* Theory development
Diagnosis, nursing, 166–167, 197
Dialogue, 198
  understanding and, 13
Dickoff and James' definition of theory development, 41, 68–70
Differentiation
  of similar concepts, 161–165
  structural idea form of, 116, 117
Dimensions of knowing, 7
  creative, 7, 197
  expressive, 199
Direct observation, 198
Direction in theory, evolving, 51–54
Discipline, 198
  nursing as, 46–48
  of nursing process, 177–178
Discrete components, structural idea form of, 116
Diversity, cultural care, 188–189
Dock's contributions to nursing theory development, 37–38
Dynamic nurse-patient relationship, 177–178

E

Early nursing models, 41–46
  health in, 45–46
  nature of nursing in, 41–42

Early nursing models—cont'd
  person in, 42–44
  society and environment in, 45
Education, nursing theory development and, 38–39
Ego as concept, 60
Ellis' definition of theory, 71
Emergence of theory, 33–56; *see also* Theory, emergence of
Emerging relationships, empirically grounded, 99–100
Empathy, 165
Empiric-abstract continuum, 59, 198
Empiric concepts, 198; *see also* Empirics
  abstract concept and, 58–60
Empiric indicators, 198; *see also* Empirics
  explicating, 100–101
  identification of, 163–164
Empiric testing, 198
Empiric theory, 198
Empirically grounded emerging relationships, 99–100
Empirics, 7–8
  knowing and, 7–8
  nursing theory as expression of, 19–31
    creation of, 26–30
    definition in, 20–21
    development processes for, 30–31
    uses of, 21–26
  patterns gone wild and, 15
Engaging in esthetics, 10–11
Environment
  in early nursing models, 45
  man and, 193–194
  relationship of individual to, 115
Envisioning in esthetics, 11
Esthetics, 10–11
  engaging in, 10–11
  envisioning in, 11
  interpreting in, 11
  knowing and, 10–11
  patterns gone wild and, 15
Ethical theory, 199
Ethics, 8–9, 199
  guidelines for, 198
  knowing and, 8–9
  patterns gone wild and, 15
  principles of, 198
  in theory-linked research, 145
Evidence in determining theory usefulness, 170
Experience, 80

Explanations
  in determining theory usefulness, 169–170
  in empirics, 8
Explanatory relationships, 199
Expression of knowledge, 5–6
Expressive dimensions of knowing, 7, 199

F

Fact, 75, 199
Features of theory, definitions and, 73
Field observation, 147
Form, structural; *see* Structure
Formal method of study, 104
Format, 64
Foundational to dependent structural idea
     form, 116
Framework
  conceptual, 197
  theoretic, 203
Function in nursing, 177–178
Functional influence, 171
Functional outcomes, 172

G

General definition, 199
Generality of theory, 131–135, 199
  research development and, 158
Generality trait, 199
Generation of theoretic relationships, 28,
  199
Goal congruence, 168–169
Grand theory, 123, 199
Grounded theory, 147, 199

H

Hall's theory
  of health, 46
  of nursing, 38, 179–180
Health
  as expanding consciousness, 191–192
  Neuman's theory of, 191–192
Health in early nursing models, 45–46
Henderson's theory
  of health, 46
  of nursing, 180
  of person, 44
Hermeneutic method of inquiry, 48
History
  nursing theory, 34–41
    borrowing from other disciplines in, 40–
     41
    conceptual models of, 39–40

History—cont'd
  nursing theory—cont'd
    development within discipline of, 41
    philosophies of practice in, 39–40
  in theory development, 28
Holism, 199
  as key nursing concept, 47–48
Holistic theory, 199
Homeodynamics, 60
Human science, 3–4
Hypothesis, 199

I

Idea
  structural clarity of, 132–133
  structural form of, 116, 117
    discrete components in, 116
    foundational to dependent, 116
Identification
  of new concepts, 165–166
  of nursing diagnosis criteria, 166–167
Identity
  professional, 22–23
  self, 23
Importance, 200
  of theory, 136–137
Inappropriate use of theories, 144
Indirect observation, 200
Individual-environment relationships, 115
Induction, 200
Inductive logic, 65–67, 200
  deduction versus, 67–68
Inductive research, 200
Influence, functional, 171
Integration, 200
  of patterns of knowing, 11–15
Interpersonal aspects of nursing, 181
Interpersonal relations in nursing, 176
Interpreting in esthetics, 11
Interpretive summary of nursing models; *see*
    Nursing conceptual model
Intervening concepts, conceptual meaning
    and, 95
Invention, 68–69
Isolated research, 200
  theory-linked research versus, 142–145

J

Johnson's theory of nursing, 192–193
Justification, 200
  understanding and, 13

Index

K

Kerlinger's view of knowing, 2–3
King's theory
  of nursing, 184–185
  of person, 44
Knower, 3
Knowing, 5, 200
  dimensions of, 7
    creative, 7, 197
    expressive, 199
  holistic view of, 4
  integration of, 6, 11–15
  patterns of, 1–17
    empirics and, 7–8
    esthetics and, 10–11
    ethics and, 8–9
    integration of, 14–15
    patterns gone wild and, 15–16
    personal knowing and, 9–10
    processes in, 2–4
    understanding and, 11–14
    wholeness in, 5–11
  personal, 9–10, 201
    patterns gone wild and, 15
  processes of, 2–4
    Western, 2
  wholeness of, 5–11
    empirics and, 7–8
    esthetics and, 10–11
    ethics and, 8–9
    personal knowing and, 9–10
Knowledge, 5, 200
  body of, 2
  ethics as moral, 8–9
  expression of, 5–6
  knower of, 3
  theory research spiral of, 146

L

Language, 82
Law, 200
  deductive reasoning and, 65
Leininger's theory of nursing, 188–189
Levine's theory
  of health, 46
  of nursing, 43, 181–182
  of society and environment, 45
Linear time, 95
Literature
  as data source, 88
  professional, 89
  research development and, 151–153

Logic, 200
  deductive, 64–65, 200
  inductive, 65–67, 200

M

Macro theory, 200
Man-living-health theory, 193–194
Martin's theory of nursing, 177
Matheney's theory of nursing, 177
McKay's definition of theory, 63–68
Meaning, conceptual; *see* Conceptual
    meaning
Medical care system in U.S., 35–36
Meta theory, 123, 200
Method, research, 153–158
Micro theory, 200
Midrange theory, 200
Mind versus body, 4
Moccia's methods for developing nursing
    knowledge, 47–48
Model, 75–76, 200–201
  conceptual; *see* Conceptual model
  early nursing; *see* Early nursing models
  theoretic, 203
Model cases as data source, 85–86
Molar theory, 201
Molecular theory, 201
Moral knowledge, ethics as, 8–9
Music as data source, 88–89

N

Nature of nursing, 41–42, 180
Neuman's theory
  of health, 191–192
  of nursing, 185–186
Newman's holistic approach, 48
Newman's theory
  of health, 46
  of nursing, 191–192
Nightingale, Florence
  development of nursing theory and, 34–35
  nursing knowledge since, 2
  society and environment theoretical ideas
    and, 45
Nurse-patient relationship, dynamic, 177–178
Nurse satisfaction in determining theory
    usefulness, 172
Nursing
  adaptation model of, 187
  behavioral system model for, 192–193
  concepts of practice of, 183–184

Nursing—cont'd
  conservation principles of, 181–182
  as helping art, 178–179
  interpersonal aspects of, 176, 181
  man-living-health theory of, 193–194
  nature of, 41–42, 180
  paradigm for, 182–183
  patient-centered approaches to, 177
  science of unitary man and, 182–183
  systems of, 184–185
  theory development in, 191–192
  theory for, 184–185
  transcultural, 188–189
Nursing care, quality and, 179–180
Nursing conceptual model; *see* Conceptual
  model; Theory
Nursing diagnosis, criteria for, 166–167,
  197
Nursing models, early; *see* Early nursing
  models
Nursing practice; *see* Practice
Nursing process, discipline and teaching of,
  177–178
Nursing Research, 39
Nursing science, paradigms, theories, and
  critiques of, 193–194
Nursing theory; *see* Theory

O

Objectivity, 201
Observation
  direct, 198
  indirect, 200
Opening in personal knowing, 9–10
Operational definition, 201
Orem's theory
  of health, 46
  of nursing, 183–184
  of person, 44
Orlando's theory of nursing, 43, 177–178
Outcomes
  determination of, 103–104
  functional, 172
  quality of life, 173
  quality-related, 171–172

P

Pain management, communication and, 25
Paradigm, 76, 201
  man-environment simultaneity, 193–194
  for nursing, 182–183

Parse's theory of nursing, 193–194
Parsimony, 134, 201
Paterson's theory
  of health, 46
  of nursing, 188
Patient-centered approaches to nursing, 177
Patient problems, total person approach to,
  185–186
Patterns
  gone wild, 15–16, 201
  of knowing, 1–17; *see also* Knowing,
  patterns of
People as data source, 89
Peplau's theory of nursing, 43, 176–177
Perceived quality of care, 172
Person
  in early nursing models, 42–44
  holistic, 47
  theoretic view of, 42–44
Personal knowing, 9–10, 201
  patterns gone wild and, 15
Phenomenology, 147
  inquiry method and, 48
Phenomenon of caring, 188–189
Philosophy, 75, 201
  of human caring, 189–191
  of practice in history of nursing theory,
  39–40
Political process of understanding, 12
Practice, 161–173, 201
  conceptual meaning and, 163–167
  deliberative application of theory and, 167
  philosophy of, in history of nursing theory,
  39–40
  theory usefulness for, 167–173
  context congruence and, 169
  explanations and, 169–170
  functional influence and, 171
  functional outcomes and, 172
  goal congruence and, 168–169
  nurse satisfaction and, 172
  perceived quality of care and, 172
  professional standards of care and, 172
  quality of life outcomes and, 173
  quality-related outcomes and, 171–172
  research evidence and, 170
  variable similarity and, 169
  theory versus, 4, 22
Predicting in empirics, 8
Predictive relationships, 201
Premises, 201
  deductive reasoning and, 65

Index

Principles, 177–178, 201
  conservation, 181–182
Problems
  research development and, 149–151
  total person approach to patient, 185–186
Processes
  for forming understanding, 201
  in nursing, 177–178
  of theory development, 27–28, 201–202
Profession, 202
Professional communication, 25–26
Professional identity, 22–23
Professional literature, 89
Propositions, 202
  deductive reasoning and, 65
Purpose, 108, 109–111, 202
  clarification of, 84
  coherence of, 23–24
  description and, 109–111
  Dickoff and James' definition of, 68

Q

Quadrant lines, 28–29
Quality
  of care as perceived, 172
  of life, 173
  nursing care and, 179–180
  outcomes related to, 171–172
Questions in theory descriptions, 109–120
  assumptions and, 118–119
  concepts and, 111–112
  definition and, 112–113
  nature of relationships and, 113–114
  purpose and, 109–111
  structure and, 111–118

R

Realization in personal knowing, 10
Reductionism, 202
Reflection, 202
  critical; *see* Critical reflection
  understanding and, 13
Related cases as data source, 87
Relationships, 202
  descriptive, 198
  dynamic nurse-patient, 177–178
  empiric methods and validation of, 101–102
  empirically grounded emerging, 99–100
  explanatory, 199

Relationships—cont'd
  generation and testing of theoretic, 28, 99–102
  of individual to environment, 115
  interpersonal, in nursing, 176, 181
  nature of, 113–114
  predictive, 201
  statements of, 202
    designing of, 98–99
  of theory, 108, 113–114
Replication, 202
  understanding and, 13
Research, 75, 141–159, 202
  in determining theory usefulness for practice, 170
  development of, 149–158
    generalizability of, 158
    literature review and, 151–153
    methods and, 153–158
    problems and, 149–151
  inductive, 200
  isolated, 200
    theory-linked versus, 142–145
  methods in, 153–158
  spiral of knowledge and, 146
  theory-generating, 145–148
  theory-linked, 145–149, 203
    comparison of components of, 150
    design of, 155–156
    isolated versus, 142–145
    problems of, 143–145
  theory-testing, 148–149
Resources in theory development, 50–51
Response, 202
  understanding and, 13
Rogers' theory
  of nursing, 182–183
  of person, 44
Roy's theory
  of health, 46
  of nursing, 187
  of society and environment, 45

S

Sample selection, 154–155
Sanger's theory of nursing, 37
Satisfaction of nurse in determining theory usefulness, 172
Science, 74–75, 202
  in development of nursing theory, 38
  human, 3–4

Index

Science—cont'd
  as method of knowing, 2–3
  of nursing, 7–8
  of unitary man, 182–183
Scientific theory ideals, 8
Scope
  classification of, 124
  theory description and, 120–125
Self esteem, 60
Self identity, 23
Semantics
  clarity and, 130–131
  consistency and, 131–132
Simplicity, 203
  critical reflection and, 133–134
Social/political process of understanding, 12
Society in early nursing models, 45
Sociopolitical process, 203
  understanding and, 12
Sound research development, 149–158; *see also* Research, development of
Specific definition, 203
Spiral of knowledge, 146
Structure, 203
  clarity of, 132–133
  consistency in, 133
  idea, 116
    broad to specific, 116
    complex to simple, 116
    discrete components and, 116
    foundational to dependent, 116
  for individual-environment relationships, 115
  theory, 108, 111–118
    assumptions and, 96–97
    clarifying context in, 97
    concepts and, 94–96
    definition of, 28, 203
    description and, 114–118
    designing relationship statements in, 98–99
    development of, 93–99
Study, formal method of, 104
Systematic abstraction, 20–21
Systems
  behavioral, as model for nursing, 192–193
  nursing, 184–185
    Neuman model of, 185–186

T

Teaching of nursing process, 177–178
Tenacity, 2–3

Testing
  empiric, 198
  of theoretic relationships, 28, 199
Theorem, 203; *see also* Theory
  deductive reasoning and, 65
Theoretic definition, 203
Theoretic framework, 203
Theoretic ideas
  about health, 45–46
  about nursing, 43
  about person, 44
  about society and environment, 45
Theoretic model, 203
Theoretic relationships, generation and testing of, 28, 99–102
Theory; *see also* Conceptual model
  armchair, 196
  atomistic, 196
  as barrier, 144–145
  borrowing of, from other disciplines, 40–41
  classification of, 124
  coherence of purpose and, 23–24
  comparative analysis of, 62–71
    Dickoff and James' definition in, 68–70
    Ellis' definition in, 71
    McKay's definition in, 63–68
    Watson's definition in, 70–71
  components of, 108–109, 197
  comprehensive definition of, 72
  concept of, 57–77, 108, 111–112; *see also* Concept
  contextualizing of; *see* Contextualizing of theory
  creation of, 26–30
  critical reflection of, 127–139; *see also* Critical reflection
  data sources for; *see* Data, sources of
  definition of, 20–21, 108, 112–113, 203
    Dickoff and James', 68–70
    Ellis', 71
    features of theory and, 73
    McKay's, 63–68
    nursing and, 71–73
    Watson's, 70–71
  deliberative application of, 28, 102–104, 198
  description of, 107–126
    assumptions in, 118–119
    components of, 108–109
    concepts in, 111–112
    definition of concepts in, 112–113

Index

Theory—cont'd
  definition of concepts in—cont'd
    guide for, 121–122
    nature of relationships in, 113–114
    purpose in, 109–111
    questions in, 109–120
    scope and, 120–125
    structure in, 114–118
  development of, 79–105; *see also* Theory
    development
  emergence of, 33–56
    contexts of, 48–51
    discipline of nursing and, 46–48
    early nursing models and, 41–46; *see
     also* Early nursing models
    evolving directions in, 51–54
    history of development of, 34–41
  as empirics; *see* Empirics
  ethical, 199
  generality of, 134–135
  grand, 123
  grounded, 147, 199
  of human caring, 189–191
  importance of, 136–137
  inappropriate use of, 144
  macro, 200
  man-living-health, 193–194
  medical care system in U.S. and, 35–36
  meta, 123
  micro, 200
  midrange, 200
  molar, 201
  molecular, 201
  practice and, 4, 22, 161–173; *see also*
    Practice
  professional communication and, 25–26
  professional identity and, 22–23
  purpose of; *see* Purpose
  research and, 141–159; *see also* Research
  scientific, 8
  systems framework for, 184–185
  uses of, 21–26; *see also* Uses of theory
  Watson's definition of, 70
Theory development, 191–192
  assumptions and, 96–97
  clarifying context and, 97
  concepts and, 94–96
  conceptual meaning in, 80–93; *see also*
    Conceptual meaning
  deliberative application of, 102–104
  designing relationship statements in, 98–
    99

Theory development—cont'd
  history of, 34–41; *see also* History, nursing
    theory
  McKay's form of, 63–68
  process of, 27–28, 30–31, 201–202
    overlap between professions and, 29
  resources and, 49
  structuring and contextualizing in, 93–99
  theoretic relationships in, 99–102
  values and, 49
Theory-generating research, 145–148
Theory-linked research; *see* Research, theory-
  linked
Time, linear, 95
Total person approach to patient problems,
  185–186
Tradition in development of nursing theory,
  36–37
Transcultural nursing, 188–189
Travelbee's theory
  of nursing, 181
  of person, 44
  of society and environment, 45
Trophicogenic as concept, 60

U

Understanding, 11
  of concept, 61–62
  formation of, 12
  patterns of knowing and, 11–14
  processes for forming, 201
Unitary man, science of, 182–183
Universality of cultural care, 188–189
Uses of theory, 21–26
  coherence of purpose and, 23–24
  kinds of, 26
  professional communication and, 25–26
  professional identity and, 22–23

V

Validation, 203
  of relationships by empiric methods, 101–
    102
  understanding and, 13
Values, theory development and, 48–50, 89–
  90
Valuing in ethics, 9
Variable similarity in determining theory
  usefulness, 169
Visual images as data source, 88

Index

W

Wald's contribution to nursing theory
    development, 37
Watson's definition of theory, 70–71
Watson's theory of nursing, 189–191
Wave lines in illustration of theory
    development, 28
Wholism; *see* Holism
Wiedenbach's theory of nursing, 43, 178–
    179

Wrubel's phenomenologic/hermeneutic
    method of inquiry, 48
Wrubel's theory of person, 44

Z

Zderad's theory
    of health, 46
    of nursing, 188